Exceptional Longevity: From Prehistory to the Present

MONOGRAPHS ON POPULATION AGING

General Editors
Bernard Jeune and James W. Vaupel

Vol. 1
Development of Oldest-Old Mortality, 1950-1990:
Evidence from 28 Developed Countries
Väinö Kannisto

Vol. 2
Exceptional Longevity: From Prehistory to the Present
Bernard Jeune and James W. Vaupel (Eds.)

Aging Research Unit
Centre for Health and Social Policy
Odense University

Exceptional Longevity:
From Prehistory to the Present

Bernard Jeune and James W. Vaupel (Eds.)

Monographs on Population Aging, 2.
Odense University Press

Exceptional Longevity: From Prehistory to the Present
© Bernard Jeune, James W. Vaupel and
Odense University Press, 1995

Printed in Denmark by Special-Trykkeriet Viborg a-s
Cover illustration: Christian Jacobsen Drakenberg (1626?-1772
ISBN 87-7838-135-5
ISBN 0909-119X

Odense University Press
55, Campusvej DK - 5230 Odense M
Tlf. +45 66 15 79 99 Fax. +45 66 15 81 26

Contents

Preface
J.W. Vaupel 9

In Search of the First Centenarians
B. Jeune 11

The Evolution of Human Longevity from the Mesolithic
to the Middle Ages: An Analysis Based on Skeletal Data
J.L. Boldsen and *R.R. Paine* 25

Patterns of Advanced Age Mortality in the Medieval Village Tirup
J.L. Boldsen 37

Alleged Danish Centenarians before 1800
T. Kjærgaard 47

Danish Centenarians after 1800
A. Skytthe and *B. Jeune* 55

Record Longevity in Swedish Cohorts Born since 1700
H. Lundström 67

The Oldest Old in Pre-Industrial Britain: Centenarians before 1800 -
Fact or Fiction?
J. Hynes 75

Record Longevity in Chinese History - Evidence from the
Wang Genealogy
Z. Zhao 93

The Emergence and Proliferation of Centenarians
J.W. Vaupel and *B. Jeune* 109

A Note on Some Historical Data on Old Age Mortality
A.R. Thatcher 117

The Earliest Centenarians: A Statistical Analysis
J.R. Wilmoth 125

Contributors

Boldsen, J.L.
    Centre for Health and Social Policy, Odense University
    Winsløwparken 17, DK-5000 Odense C
    Denmark

Hynes, J.
    41 Roe Lane, Kingsbury
    London NW9 9BB
    England

Jeune, B.
    Centre for Health and Social Policy, Odense University
    Winsløwparken 17, DK-5000 Odense C
    Denmark

Kjærgaard, T.
    The National History Museum at Frederiksborg
    DK-3400 Hillerød
    Denmark

Lundström, H.
    Statistiska Centralbyrån
    S-11581 Stockholm
    Sweden

Paine, R.R.
    McMicken College of Arts and Sciences, Dept. of Anthropology
    University of Cincinnati, P.O. Box 210380
    Cincinnati OH 45221-0380, USA

Skytthe, A.
    Centre for Health and Social Policy, Odense University
    Winsløwparken 17, DK-5000 Odense C
    Denmark

Thatcher, A.R.
    129 Thetford Road, New Malden
    Surrey KT3 5DS
    England

Vaupel, J.W.
    Centre for Health and Social Policy, Odense University
    Winsløwparken 17, DK-5000 Odense C
    Denmark

Wilmoth, J.R.
    Department of Demography, University of California
    2232 Piedmont Avenue
    Berkeley CA 94720, USA

Zhao, Z.
    School of Sociology, University of New South Wales
    Kensington, Sydney 2052
    Australia

Preface

The storied realms of exceptional longevity were scrutinized at a research workshop held at Hindsgavl, Denmark, in September 1994. The vast majority of reputed centenarians in the past, and most in most countries even today, lived less than 100 years. On the other hand, the number of genuine longlivers is exploding and a substantial proportion of current newborns in developed countries may survive to celebrate their 100th birthdays. Extremely few of our grandparents endured a century but centenarians may be commonplace among our grandchildren. Research of the caliber presented at the Hindsgavl workshop - melding judicious scepticism and painstaking scholarship with intellectual excitement about the advancing frontier of survival - is warranted.

The Hindsgavl workshop, which was supported by grants from the Danish Research Councils, the U.S. National Institute on Aging, and the Wellcome Trust, led to this monograph. Most of the chapters are revised versions of papers presented at the workshop. Others, including Wilmoth's impressive analysis of when the first centenarians might have lived and Boldsen's suggestive findings about the very high levels of mortality at older ages in medieval Denmark, were motivated by controversy fanned at the workshop. The first flames of the controversy were sparked by the historical research of the project on the Maximal Length of Life led by Peter Laslett of Trinity College, Cambridge University, and by the incendiary hypothesis of Bernard Jeune that there were no true centenarians before 1800 and no true supercentenarians (110+) before 1950 in any population or period of history.

Only a fraction of the participants in the workshop are authors of chapters in this monograph; many others made important contributions that are reflected here. In addition to Peter Laslett, Michel Allard, Otto Andersen, Edit Beregi, James Curtsinger, Claudio Franceschi, Bo Hagberg, Shiro Horiuchi, Väinö Kannisto, Niels Keiding, Henning Kirk, J.A. Louhija, Jay Olshansky, Thomas Perls, Karen Ritchie, Jean-Marie Robine, Sven-Mårten Samuelsson, Marianne Schroll, Thorkild Sørensen, Richard Suzman, Andrus Viidik, Frans Willekens, and Anatoli Yashin, among others, helped enrich the discussion of longevity. Exceptional longevity was one topic at the Hindsgavl workshop; other topics included the health characteristics of centenarians, studies of elderly twins, and methods for analyzing data on twins and centenarians: various participants, in addition to those listed above, played active roles in these other sessions. Lise Stark, who with Lis Bluhme helped manage the workshop, produced the typescript for the monograph. Axel Skytthe, Kirill Andreev, Ivan Iachine, and Wang Zhenglian provided technical assistance. A grant from the Danish Research Councils enabled publication. Bernard Jeune and I are responsible for errors.

Professor James W. Vaupel

In Search of the First Centenarians

by Bernard Jeune

It is amazing that most literature on longevity and centenarians is based on *the hypothesis of a secret of longevity*, which can be summarized in the following four allegations:
1. maximum life-span is fixed
2. longevity is genetically determined
3. centenarians have always existed
4. centenarians are qualitatively different.

In my opinion each allegation is debatable. Some evidence that does not support them will be presented in this monograph. I have therefore proposed an alternative hypothesis, which I call *the secret of tails* (Jeune 1994). According to this hypothesis we can consider the proliferation of centenarians, which is a significant feature of actual demographic aging (Kannisto 1994, Vaupel and Jeune 1994), as a new historical phenomenon due to a demographic shift to the right of the extreme tail of the survivorship distribution, which is not due to any other secret than the factors involved in this shift to the right.

As such the present proliferation of centenarians and the emergence of supercentenarians, which is the result of this proliferation, does not support the first allegation of the dominant hypothesis. To a certain degree this shift to the right of the extreme tail does not support the second allegation either. In the concept of "genetic determination" longevity is considered to be pre-programmed in the genes. It thereby eliminates any substantial impact of the environment. However, heritability of longevity has been estimated to be 0.2-0.3 and the heritability of frailty to be 0.5 in a Danish twin population (McGue et al. 1993, Herskind et al. 1994, Yashin and Iachine 1994). The interplay between genes and environment is better reflected in the concept of "genetic regulation", which is included in the adaptivity hypothesis (Franceschi et al. 1991). This hypothesis seems more in accordance with a secret of tails than a secret of longevity.

Assuming a secret of longevity, centenarians might always have existed, independently of the size of the population and the level of mortality. Therefore, if this is not the case, it would be in favour of the alternative hypothesis. The same would be the case if some special traits distinctly characterized centenarians which is almost a tenet in centenarian research, and vice versa.

The question - have centenarians always existed? - is therefore not only of interest to historians. It is also an important question for gerontologists. With reference to the well-known novel by Proust ("A la recherche du temps perdu"), I have proposed the title "In search of the first centenarians" for research which can contribute to the answering of this question. For the purpose of studying this question without any prejudice I have also deliberately claimed that supercentenarians did not exist before 1950 and centenarians not before 1800 in any population and in any period of world history (Jeune 1993, 1994).

I shall not here present all my arguments for this working hypothesis. Let me only refer to the work of Vincent (1951), who analysed the most valid data on the mortality of oldest-old people he could get from the first half of this century (data from four European countries). On this basis he found it very improbable that even one individual "in the actual conditions" could reach an age beyond 110 years. Let me also refer to the work of Thoms (1873) in which he refuted most of the reported centenarians in England and Wales around 1870. Overreporting of age in this country with a long tradition of good vital statistics was in the late 1800s in fact not a minor problem but almost the rule.

To start a very time-consuming historical, demographic work on the basis of the alternative hypothesis might be considered to be useless or even nonsense. However, regarding the impact of the old myths on longevity in scientific literature, including the strong preservation of Buffon's concept of a fixed maximum life-span in most introductions to gerontological textbooks, it seems justifiable to investigate this question. Such work could contribute further to a better understanding of the evolution of the interplay between genes and the environment. But, as it is evident from the contributions to this monograph, it is not an easy task to investigate whether supercentenarians have existed before 1950 or centenarians before 1800.

Kannisto (1994) has recently shown that a proliferation of oldest-old people has taken place in recent decades. As shown in the following table, in developed countries with reliable data centenarians have increased twentyfold since 1960, and the proportion has increased from about 0.5 to nearly 5 per 100,000. This proliferation of centenarians is also visible in Denmark, as shown in the following figure.

As suggested by Skytthe and Jeune in this monograph it seems improbable that centenarians existed in Denmark before 1800 or at least exceptionally few existed before that date. Also in Sweden centenarians before that date seem to be very rare (Wilmoth and Lundström 1995 and Lundström in this monograph). However, the Danish population was very small at that time - less than 1 million. It reached 1 million some years after 1800.

PROPORTION OF CENTENARIANS IN TOTAL POPULATION, 1960 AND 1990

Country	1.1.1960		1.1.1990	
	Number	Per million	Number	Per million
Austria	25	3.5	232	29.8
Belgium	...	...	474	48.1
Denmark	19	4.1	323	62.8
England & Wales	531	11.6	3890	76.3
Estonia	...	...	42	26.7
Finland	11	2.5	141	28.3
France	371	8.1	3853	67.9
Germany, West	119	2.2	2528	40.0
Iceland	3	17.0	17	66.7
Ireland	...	...	87	24.8
Italy	265	5.4	2047	35.5
Japan	155	1.7	3126	25.3
Netherlands	62	5.4	818	54.7
New Zealand	18	7.6	198	59.2
Norway	73	20.4	300	70.7
Portugal	...	...	268	27.2
Singapore	...	...	41	15.2
Sweden	72	9.6	583	68.1
Switzerland	29	5.4	338	50.4
14 countries	1753	5.3	18394	45.1
19 countries	...	...	19306	44.3

Nevertheless, the reported number and proportion of centenarians in Denmark was much higher in the first half of the 1800s than later in the 1800s (see Skythe and Jeune in this monograph), and much higher in Sweden in the later half of the 1700s than in the first half of the 1800s (see Lundström in this monograph). The reported decline of Danish centenarians in the 1800s could either be due to a dramatic deterioration of oldest-old mortality or be an artefact of substantial age-exaggeration. The latter explanation is the most plausible.

The history of exceptional longevity reveals an even more dramatic decline. If we were to believe what is reported in ancient literature, it is obvious that the Deluge swept away the pluricentenarians. Ernest (1938) mentioned that the semi-divine persons of the Hindu Sagas lived hundred of thousands of years, and that on

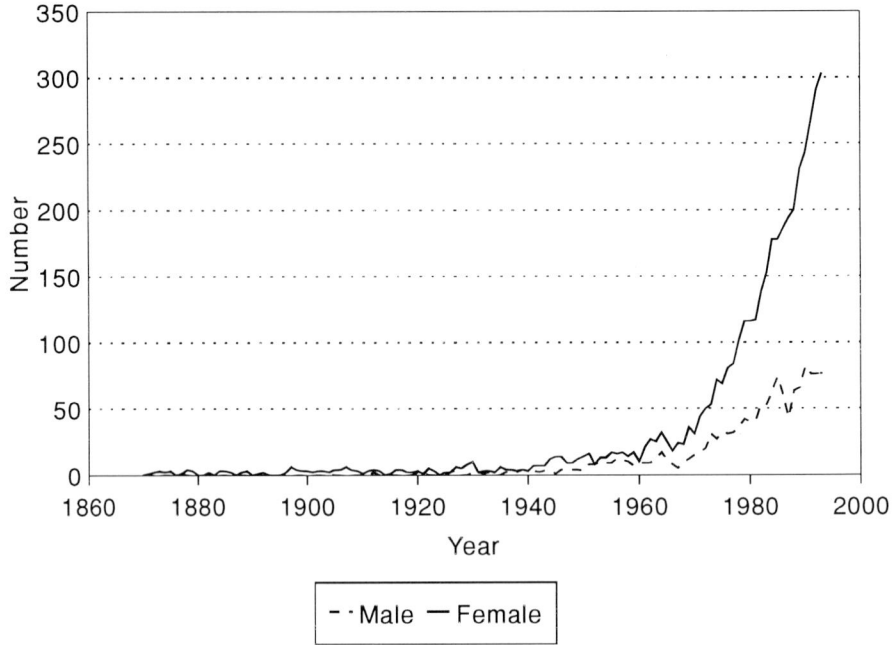

Figure 1. Number of Centenarians in Denmark.

average each of ten rulers of Ancient Babylon lived about 43,000 years. The antediluvian patriarchs lived almost 1,000 years (Adam 930 years, Seth 912 years, Jared 962 years, Enoch 965 years, Lamech 777 years and the oldest: Methuselah 969 years). Noah, who survived the Deluge, reached the age of 950 years.

Among the postdiluvian supercentenarians who are mentioned in Genesis the males from Noah to Abraham lived almost 300 years (Abraham himself reached the age of 275 years). And after Abraham the supercentenarians did not reach higher ages than famous reported supercentenarians from modern historic time: Sarah 127 years, Ismail 137 years, Isaac 180 years, Jacob 147 years, Joseph 110 years, Moses 120 years, Aaron 110 years.

More realistic perhaps is the declaration in Psalm 90: "The days of our age are threescore years and ten, and though men be so strong that they come to fourscore years....". This could very well have been true until recently. Although Lucian of Samosata in an epistle from the reign of Marcus Aurelius (about 150 A.D.) mentioned 27 kings, 17 philosophers, 3 historians and 4 literati as centenarians, Montagu (1994), who has written a paper on the length of life among the oldest Greeks and Romans mentioned in the Oxford Classical Dictionary, only regarded 10 males as "firmly" over 80 years (Thatcher, personal communication). Although in modern literature Gorgias of Leontium is often reported to be 107 years, none of those in whom

Montagu believed were over 100 years old.

Ernest (1938) stressed that "no one appears to have been sufficiently interested in longevity to compile a list of longlivers" from Lucian until the 16th century. I have not found anybody who has commented on the authenticity of such reported supercentenarian medieval saints as St. Mungo of Glagow (185 years) and St. Patrick of Ireland (122 years). Some interesting findings from the medieval period in Europe and China are presented in this monograph (see the contribution by Boldsen and by Zhao). Although, these authors draw different conclusions on the possibilities of centenarians, nothing in their findings suggests that ages higher than 110 years (supercentenarian) were possible in the medieval period.

However, even scholars as respected as Bacon and Haller believed in some of these supercentenarians from the ancient and medieval periods. Haller mentioned more than a thousand centenarians and more than hundred supercentenarians in the last volume of his "Elementa physiologiae corporis humani" (1760). He believed that it would be possible to reach the age of 200 years.

In the same period Buffon (1760/1835) stated that "l'homme qui ne meurt point de maladies accidentelles vit partout quatre-vingt-dix ou cent ans" ("the man who does not die of incidental diseases reaches everywhere the age of ninety or one hundred years"). He introduced the concept of a fixed maximum life-span depending on the duration of growth, which was specific for each species, and stressed that nothing could change what he called "the fixed laws which regulate the number of years". However, this new concept had no impact on the torrent of catalogues on longlivers which appeared in the late 1700s and especially in the 1800s. The Danish gallery by Luxdorph is presented in this monograph (Kjærgaard).

For many years the most famous and venerated supercentenarians have been largely accepted as supercentenarians. The story of some of these mostly poor persons like Parr and Drakenberg turned into legends. Many countries have had their famous centenarians. In England, besides "old, old, very old Parr", there were Catherine of Desmonde and Henry Jenkins. In Denmark, besides the famous seaman Drakenberg, there was Peter Henricson, who was known from the well-preserved epitaphe in the church of a small town, Møgeltønder, and Live Livsdatter, who was the servant of the Danish scientist Thycho Brahe. In Sweden there was Jon Andersson who even surpassed the age of Drakenberg. In USA there was Joice Heth, who was the nurse of George Washington, Yarrow Mamout, who was known as the "chukling old negro", Christopher Vanpool, who was known as "the durable Dutchman" and Samuel Mecutcheon, who was known as the oldest citizen of Philadelphia. John and Sarah Rovin are the most famous Hungarian supercentenarians. The Canadian supercentenarian, Pierre Joubert, is the only one in

CATALOGUES OF LONGLIVERS

NEWTON, Thomas: The Worthye Books of Old Age (London 1569).

BACON, Francis (1561-1626): The History of Life and Death (London, 1638).

COMMIERS, C de.: La médicine universelle, ou l'art de se conserver en santé et de prolonger la vie (Paris 1687).

LONGEVILLE, Harcouët de.: Histoire des personnes qui ont vécu plusieurs siècles (Paris 1715).

ANONYMOUS: Almanach de la Viellesse, ou Notice de tous ceux qui ont vécu cent ans ou plus (Paris 1756).

LOTTIN, Augustin-Martin: Almanach des centenaires (10 vol., Paris, 1764-1771)

HALLER, Albrecht von (1708-1777): Elementa physiologiae corporis humani (In the last of 8 volumes, 1757-1760).

LUXDORPH, Bolle Willum (1716-1788): Catalogus longaevorum (Copenhagen, 1780).

EASTON, James: Human Longevity (Salisbury, 1799).

SCHROETER, J.S.: Das Alter und die untrüglichen Mittel alt zu werden, nebst 11790 Beispielen von Personen, welsche 80 bis 190 Jahre alt geworden sind (Berlin, 1805).

SINCLAIR, Sir John: The Code on Health and Longevity (Edinburgh, 1807).

RUSH, Benjamin: Medical Inquiries and Observations on Old Age (Vol. 2, Philadelphia, 1809)

TAYLOR, J.: Annals of Health and Long Life with Biographical Anecdotes of 140 Persons who Attained Extreme Old Age (London, 1818).

NEUMAIR, G.A.G.: Die sichersten Mittel ein sehr hohes Alter zu erreichen, mit mehr als 7000 Beispielen von Personen, die...bis 360 Hahre alt geworden sind (Leipzig, 1822).

ANONYMOUS: An Account of Persons Remarkable for their Health and Longevity (London, 1829).

LEJONCOURT, Charles: Galeries des Centenaires, anciens et modernes (Paris, 1842).

VAN OVEN, B.: On the Decline of Life and Health and Disease, Being an Attempt to Investigate the Causes of Longevity (London, 1853).

BAILEY, T.: Records of Longevity (London, 1857).

WATSON, J.F.: Annals of Philadelphia and Pennsylvania in the Olden Time (Philadelphia, 1857)

WARE, J.R.: Famous Centenarians. Records of 200 Persons who Have Lived to be 100 Years and upwards (London, 1885).

which Young (1905) and later Bowermann (1939) believed.

Not until the second half of the 1800s did Thoms and others try to assess what was fact and what fiction. Thoms (1873, 2nd ed. 1878) not only refuted such famous reputed supercentenarians as Catherine of Desmonde, Thomas Parr and Henry Jenkins, but he also thoroughly examined reported centenarians from his own time. About 90% reported to be centenarians in the newspapers during the period 1868-72 could be refuted.

FAMOUS SUPERCENTENARIANS BEFORE 1900		
Catherine of Desmonde	1464-1604	140 years
Peter Henricson	1465-1592	127 years
Thomas Parr	1483-1635	152 years
Henry Jenkins	1501-1670	169 years
Petracz Czartan	1539-1724	185 years
Live Livsdatter	1575-1698	123 years
Jon Andersson	1582-1729	147 years
Christian Jacobsen Drakenberg	1626-1772	146 years
Joice Heth	1684->1845	>161 years
Yarrow Mamout	1685->1819	>134 years
Pierre Joubert	1701-1814	113 years
Christopher Vanpool	1754-1866	112 years
Samuel Mecutcheon	1767-1889	122 years
John and Sarah Rovin		172/164 years

Ernest (1938) mentioned that a similar high proportion of reported centenarians from the same period could not be verified in some statistical investigations from Canada, Bavaria and Prussia. Among 1756 reported centenarians at a census in Bulgaria at the begining of this century only 51 could be verified (Vischer 1945). Age-exaggeration was in fact not a minor problem around 1900 in most of Europe. Today the same is the case for most countries in the world, especially in countries with a high proportion of illiteracy. It seems that the lower life expectancy is the higher is the reported proportion of centenarians and the reported record of longevity. Age-exaggeration has been documented in the new tales of high proportions of centenarians in certain mountain areas, like Abkhasia, Kashmir and Vilcabamba in the Andes. Systematic age-exaggeration in an illiterate population began already from the age of 70 and the exaggeration increased with age to over 30 years (Mazess and Forman 1979).

As late as in the 1970s a new era of alleged 'oldest in the world' emerged. Many of them have been described in newspapers, in the Guiness Book of Records, and even in scientific journals, like the 168-year-old Shirali Muslimov from the ex-Soviet Union, the 137-year-old Charlie Smith from USA, the 127-year-old Miguel Carpio Mendieta from Vilcabamba (Ecuador), the 120-year-old Shigechiyo Izumi from Japan etc. They are typically all men.

However, in well-documented centenarian studies from the 1980's in Europe these extreme ages were never reached. The oldest well-documented person seems to be Jeanne Calment from Arles in France, who was investigated as 115 years old in the French centenarian study (Allard 1991). She is now 120 years old and certainly the best documented supercentenarian until now (Allard et al. 1994). The oldest woman in the Nordic countries seems to have been Hulda Johansson, who recently died at the age of 112. The first supercentenarian has just emerged in Denmark in November 1994, a 110-year-old woman from Jutland.

The oldest man may have been John Evans from England who died in 1990 at the age of 112 years and 9 months (Thatcher 1992). In the near future he can be surpassed by the Danish-born American, Christian Mortensen, who has the possibility of reaching the age of 113 in August 1995. In cooperation with John Wilmoth, who has done several interviews with him at a Danish nursing home near San Francisco, where he lives, Skytthe and I have collected a lot of evidence that he really is 112 years old.

Supercentenarians in fact seem to be a very new phenomenon, which first emerged among women and some years later among men. It seems unlikely that the number of supercentenarians living in the world today is beyond 100 and maybe it is only around 50. It is therefore not surprising that more sceptical demographers, like Vincent (1951) in the fifties and Kannisto until recently, did not believe in ages higher than 110 years in the given conditions (Vincent: "en l'état actuel des choses"). The question is therefore when and where this age was surpassed.

Young included no supercentenarians in whom he believed in the first edition of his book "On Centenarians" (1899), but two in the second edition (1905), and later Bowermann (1939) added four believable ones to these two, all in all six supercentenarians. The authenticity of these possible supercentenarians from before 1950 are now under investigation in Peter Laslett's group on "Maximal Length of Life" at the University of Cambridge. Some of them cannot be further investigated because the original documents have disappeared (this is for example the case with the above-mentioned Pierre Joubert), but Julia Hynes has done a thorough investigation of the Irish lady Katherine Plunket who died in 1932. Although the evidence is not conclusive if all the criteria of Thoms are applied, it cannot be refuted that she died at the age of 111.

Nevertheless, the emergence - or reemergence - of supercentenarians seems to be a very new phenomenon, made possible by the proliferation of centenarians in recent years. It therefore seems obvious to search for an explanation for this new demographic development. Is it mainly due to the number of births hundred years ago, to the decline in infant mortality and to a lesser degree also to the decline in adult mortality? This is the conventional wisdom.

Few imagine, however, that a decline in old age mortality has had any impact on this new development. It has almost been a tenet that mortality among oldest-old did not change, at least until recently as demonstrated by Kannisto (1994). However, this tenet is based on estimated mortality rates from reported data from the past century and the first half of this century, which may be distorted due to age-exaggeration.

Vaupel and Jeune (1994, see also this monograph) have shown that about 2/3 or more of the proliferation of centenarians is due to improved survival from age 80 to 100. The chance of enduring from birth to age 100 over the course of human existence may have risen from one in several million to two in hundred. If, as stated by Vaupel and Jeune in this monograph, "the chance of surviving to the age 100 is about 1 in 20 million when life expectancy is 20 and about 1 in 80,000 when life expectancy is 40 (a level not reached in Western Europe until the early 19th century), then centenarians must have been exceedingly rare in most countries before the modern era".

Furthermore, if supercentenarians first emerged when life expectancy was about 70 and the size of the world population was over 4 billion, why should centenarians have existed when life expectancy was below 40 and world population below 1 billion, especially in historical periods with no evidence of improvement in old age mortality, because nursing and treatment of elderly people were very poor and the life-styles of elderly people did not change?

At this stage of the history of longevity, I therefore find it more fruitful to discuss the conditions of falsification than to corroborate what may be a false tenet. As one says in court: "Ei incumbit probatio qui dicit non qui negat". Like Vincent, we do not have to believe it, "jusqu'a preuve contraire" and this has to be found in Thoms' "species of evidence".

However, other authors in this monograph have found evidence of true centenarians before this era. Hynes thoroughly points out "a range of difficulties which might be impossible to overcome". She therefore argues that Thoms' criteria are too strict in searching for true centenarians before 1800. This is also the reason why Skytthe and Jeune propose four levels of evidence, but some of the centenarians that Hynes accepts do not fulfil the lowest levels (D and C). Therefore, if birth and death certificates are lacking some of the evidence of life history that Hynes proposes should be incorporated in the lowest level in a strict way.

On the other hand, if birth and death certificates exist as they did in the Norwegian case investigated by Kjærgaard, but only few pieces of evidence of life history and family reconstruction are collected (level B and A), it cannot be concluded with "no doubt at all" that the same name in the birth and the death certificate in fact refers to the same person, especially when information is lacking from a thirty year period from the age of 71 years.

In the documentation of supercentenarians today we certainly also need a differentiation of the highest level (A), which concerns family reconstruction. The family reconstruction of Jeanne Calment is extremely high, because her family had lived for at least three centuries in Arles, which has an archive going back to the 17th century. The family reconstruction of Christian Mortensen is high, but does not reach the level of Jeanne Calment. In the case of Kathrine Plunket the level of family reconstruction is low, but it seems to be extremely difficult to get any further.

Totally different criteria are used in the presentation by Zhao on the Chinese Wang Genealogy, relying on other data sources than parish registers, including genealogical data using the traditional Chinese calendar, the "Nian Hao"-system, and the importance of the time of birth for a person's destiny. It could therefore be recommended that different criteria for different periods and different places be established.

Zhao also uses a demographic explanation in his arguments for the existence of centenarians before the modern era. On the basis of some historical data on old age mortality Thatcher estimates the probability of survival from age 0 to 100 for a life table cohort born in 1700. This estimate comes to about 1 in 100,000 which is consistent with the estimates of Zhao and Vaupel and Jeune.

The final contribution, by Wilmoth, is a comprehensive analysis based on a set of different assumptions, which has the great advantage of delimiting the problem. Assuming a remaining life expectancy at age 50 of about 14 years, he concludes that the emergence of centenarians "probably occurred during the time of the first great human civilizations". Wilmoth emphasizes, however, that this conclusion "is very sensitive to our assumption about the average level" of life expectancy at age 50 in the pre-industrial period. If the remaining life expectancy at this age was 12 years or lower, as Boldsen suggests it was in Medieval Denmark, centenarians seem improbable prior to the industrial period.

This monograph begins with the contribution by Boldsen and Paine on longevity from the Mesolithic to the Middle Ages based on analyses of skeleton materials. In the last chapter Wilmoth reviews the literature on population size, mortality level and life expectancy during world history. His array of alternative assumptions and estimates for different historical periods closes the monograph with a frame for further research on this topic.

Finally, I want to illustrate that the tail hypothesis was already expressed in 1865 by Lewis Caroll. The following tail poem "Fury and the mouse" from "Alice in Wonderland" was written 50 years before the French poet, Appollinaire, wrote his "calligrammes" and the French surrealists considered the author of this tail poem a precursor:

"You promised me to tell me your history, you know," said Alice...
"Mine is a long and a sad tale!" said the Mouse, turning to Alice and sighing.
"It **is** a long tail, certainly", said Alice, looking down with wonder at the Mouse's tail; "but why do you call it sad?"
And she kept on puzzling about it while the Mouse was speaking, so that her idea of the tale was something like this: (see poem overleaf).

"You are not attending!" said the Mouse to Alice severely. "What are you thinking of?"
"I beg your pardon", said Alice very humbly: "you had got to the fifth bend I think?"
"I had **not**!" cried the Mouse angrily.
"A knot!" said Alice, always ready to make herself useful, and looking anxiously about her. "Oh, do let me help to undo it!"
"I shall do nothing of the sort," said the Mouse, getting up and walking away. "You insult me by talking such nonsense!".

The poem is not merely a tale but a tale in a tail. I think that it is a good model for exploring the question of longevity. It is clear from this that we do not have to find a special unchanging secret of longevity but we have to keep on puzzling about the tail and its secret in a changing world.

FURY AND THE MOUSE

                    Fury said to a
                  mouse, that he
                 met in the
                house,
             "Let us
            both go
             to law:
              I will
                prosecute
                  you. Come, I'll
                     take no denial.
                   We must
                   have a trial:
                 For really
                this morning
               I've nothing
             to do".
         Said the
          mouse to the
              cur, "Such a
                 trial,
                    dear Sir,
                      With no
                     jury or
                    judge,
                would be
             wasting
            our breath".
       I'll be judge
      I'll be jury",
       Said
         cunning
           old Fury
            "I'll
              try the
             whole
            cause
          and
          condemn
          you
           to
             death".

Literature

Allard, M. 1991. A la recherche du secret des centenaires. *Le Cherche Midi Editeur*, Paris.

Allard, M., V. Lèbre, J-M. Robine. 1994. Les 120 ans de Jeanne Calment. *Le Cherche Midi Editeur*, Paris.

Bowermann, W.G. 1939. Centenarians. *Transactions of the Actuarial Society of America* 40:360-378.

Buffon. 1835. Oeuvres Complètes de Buffon. Tome IV, p. 108, *P. Duménil*, Paris.

Caroll, L. 1865. Alice's Adventures in Wonderland. New version *Wordsworth Editions Ltd.*, Ware, Hertfordshire, 1992 p. 21.

Ernest, M. 1938. The longer life. *Adam & Co.*, London.

Franceschi, C., D. Monti, A. Cossariza, F. Fagnoni, G. Passeri, P. Sansoni. 1991. Aging, longevity and cancer: studies in Down's syndrome and centenarians. *Ann NY Acad Sci* 621:428-440.

Herskind, A.M., M. McGue, N.V. Holm, B. Harvald. 1994. How heritable is human longevity. A population based study of 2803 Danish twin pairs. Manuscript, Odense University.

Jeune, B. 1993. Centenarians - tail or tale? Presentation at the 46th Annual Scientific Meeting of The Gerontological Society of America, New Orleans, November 19-23, 1993. Manuscript.

Jeune, B. 1994. Centenarians - tail or tale? (In Danish) *Gerontology and Society* 10(1):4-6.

Jeune, B. 1994. Morbus Centenarius or Sanitas Longaevorum? *Population Studies of Aging # 15*. Center for Health and Social Policy, Odense University, Denmark.

Kannisto, V. 1994. Development of Oldest-Old Mortality, 1950-1990: Evidence from 28 Developed Countries. *Odense Monographs on Population Aging 1*, *Odense University Press*, Odense.

Mazess, R.B., and S. Forman. 1979. Longevity and age exaggeration in Vilcabamba. *Journal of Gerontology* 34:94-98.

McGue, M., J.W. Vaupel, N.V. Holm, and B. Harvald. 1993. Longevity Is Moderately Heritable in a Sample of Danish Twins Born 1870-1880. *Journal of Gerontology* 48 (6):B237-B244.

Montagu J.D. 1994. Length of life in the ancient world: a controlled study. *Journal of the Royal Society of Medicine* 87:25-26.

Thatcher A.R. 1992. Trends in numbers and mortality at high ages in England and Wales. *Populations Studies* 46:411-426.

Thoms, W.J. 1873. Human Longevity. Its Facts and Its Fictions. *John Murray*, London.

Vaupel, J.W., and B. Jeune. 1994. The emergence and proliferation of centenarians. *Population Studies of Aging # 12*. Center for Health and Social Policy, Odense University, Denmark.

Vischer, A.L. 1945. Medizinische Betrachtungen bei einem Hundertjährigen. *Schweizerische Medizinische Wochenschrift* 75:747-748.

Vincent, P. 1951. La mortalité des vieillards. *Population*, Paris 6:181-204.

Wilmoth, J., and H. Lundström. 1995. Extreme longevity in five countries: Presentation of trends with special attention to issues of data quality. *European Journal of Population*, forthcoming.

Yashin, A.I., and I.A. Iachine. 1994. Environment determines 50% of variability in individuality frailty: Results from study of Danish twins born in 1870-1900. *Population Studies of Aging # 10*. Center for Health and Social Policy, Odense University, Denmark.

Young, T.E. 1905. On Centenarians. London.

The Evolution of Human Longevity from the Mesolithic to the Middle Ages: An Analysis Based on Skeletal Data

by Jesper L. Boldsen & Richard R. Paine

The mythology concerning human longevity in the past is extensive. The first ten men mentioned in the Bible, Adam through Noah (except Cain and Abel), lived on average more than 850 years (Genesis 5: 1-32). Methuselah lived for 969 years. This was the maximum, but by no means exceptional. However, already in antediluvian time God fixed the living day of man to 120 years. Apparently, it took some time to adjust to this standard. The mean longevity of the eight male generations from Noah to Abraham was close to 300 years. There was a clear and statistically significant tendency to decline (r=-0.88, t=4.58, df=6, p<0.001; Genesis, 11:10-26).

Until recently it was believed that people in the European Middle Ages, if they survived the hazards of infancy and childhood, lived 'as long as people do today'. Only palaeodemographic studies of large samples of skeletons representing the general population can contribute to the thorough rejection of such false assumptions (Gejvall 1960, Boldsen and Vellev 1981, Boldsen 1984 and 1988, and Boldsen, Kieffer-Olsen and Pentz 1985). However, it is only possible to conduct thorough palaeodemographic studies on recently excavated skeletons and on material from the Middle Ages. In spite of this, this chapter tries to recover information on longevity in the more distant past by utilizing skeletal material covering most of European postglacial history. In doing so we will have to make sweeping generalizations and aim at pitifully simplistic conclusions about the demography of past communities.

The original title of this chapter was: Extreme Longevity from the Mesolithic to the Middle Ages. However, there is nothing extreme about the old ages discussed in this chapter. In fact, determination of skeletal age at death is rather inaccurate in all but the youngest adults. It is only possible with available methods to estimate the fraction of the population that lived into a given anatomically defined age-related stage. This chapter presents an overview of changes of the fraction of the adult population that reached such a stage. The time period covered comprises some 8,000 years from the Mesolithic to the late Middle Ages.

Temporal frame, Material and Methods

Many students of human longevity might not be familiar with the sequence and classification of prehistoric periods in Europe. Consequently, the outlines of a temporal frame will be provided. It is hoped that this frame will help guide the reader's thoughts along the lines of the argument. The datings are in Table 1. As a biological species man was created in the Palaeolithic - a period stretching from around 2.5 million years ago to the end of the last glaciation at about 8300 BC.

Man has not remained genetically unaltered through the last 10,000 years or so, but the most important changes in this period have occurred in the socio-cultural sphere rather than in the genetic make up of our species.

The end of the last Ice Age saw the start of a new era of European history - the Mesolithic. Both the Upper Palaeolithic and the Mesolithic periods were characterised by subsistence based on foraging - gathering and hunting. Right at the end of what was the Ice Age of central and northern Europe, people in the Middle East adopted a new way of living - agriculture. They underwent the so-called Neolithic revolution. Agriculture became the dominant way of subsistence in central Europe by 5000 BC. The transition in southern Scandinavia was delayed by some 1000 years (Jensen 1988). The Mesolithic skeletons were derived from six different sites from a wider area of Europe than the skeletons from other periods. In fact, three of the samples are from Scandinavian sites (Albrethsen and Brinch Petersen 1976 and Larsson 1989). There are two samples from France and only one sample derived from a site in central Europe (Saller 1962).

The Neolithic period lasted several thousand years. Starting with the formation of small, probably only semi-sedentary tribal communities subsisting on slash and burn agriculture and a lot of gathering and hunting. It was in this period permanently socially stratified societies evolved in Europe. During the latter half of the Neolithic period the Indo-European language community and the cultures that went with it spread over the face of the continent (Mallory 1989). The boundary between the Late Stone Age and the Early Bronze Age is quite arbitrary. In Denmark it is actually defined by the appearance of special types of flint tools and not by bronze implements as such (eg Rasmussen 1990). Neolithic skeletal samples are derived from nine sites. One site from each of the countries Austria (Ehgartner 1959), Czechoslovakia (Buchvaldek and Koutecky 1970) and France (Patte 1971) and six sites from Germany (Bach 1978, Czarnetzki 1966 and Grimm 1958, 1959 and 1961).

Table 1: The temporal frame and the numbers of skeletons providing information for the analyses

Period	Dates	Skeletons	Sites
Mesolithic	10,000-4,000 BC	89	6
Neolithic	6,000-1,500 BC	418	9
Bronze Age	1,800-500 BC	419	2
Pre-Roman Iron Age	1,000-0 BC	340	6
Roman Iron Age	100 BC-AD 500	191	2
Early Middle Ages	AD 500-1050	1088	7
Late Middle Ages	AD 1050-1550	106	1
SOUTHERN SCANDINAVIAN MATERIAL			
Early Roman Iron Age	0 BC - AD 200	186	many
Late Roman Iron Age	AD 200-400	104	many
Middle Ages	AD 1000-1536	1479	6
All periods		4420	

In the Bronze Age urban communities formed in central and southern Europe. However, the majority of the population went on subsisting on agriculture. Many culturally important events took place during the Bronze Age, eg the historical events behind the narratives in much of the Old Testament and the travels of Odysseus. Like the transition from the Neolithic period to the Bronze Age the beginning of the following period, the Iron Age, was a long and slow process. The Bronze Age skeletal data come from two Austrian samples (Bertemes 1989 and Berner, no date).

Iron metallurgy was invented early in the second millennium BC. But many centuries were to pass before iron came into regular use in Europe. The Iron Age framed European classical history. The rise and fall of the Roman Empire took place during this period. But like in the Bronze Age the majority of the population went on living in small rural communities only contributing to the spectacular events of written Iron Age history by being soldiers and paying taxes. Iron age skeletons are treated in four categories: central European Pre-Roman Iron Age, central European Roman Iron Age, Danish Early Roman Iron Age and Danish Late Roman Iron Age. The central European Pre-Roman Iron Age skeletons originate from six German sites

(Spindler 1977, Schwidetzky 1978, Ehrhardt and Simon 1971, Kramer 1964 and Keiling 1974). Two central European Roman Iron Age skeletal samples are included, from Germany (no reference) and Hungary (Ery 1973). Data on all Danish Iron Age skeletons have been derived from Sellevold, Hansen and Jørgensen (1984).

The Middle Ages which followed the Iron Age was the period of universal Catholicism in central and northern Europe. In central and southern Europe the Middle Ages started at the conquest of Rome in AD 410. But in Scandinavia the Viking Age, generally considered a part of the Iron Age, lasted till around AD 1000 (Sawyer 1988). The urban communities grew during the Middle Ages and around AD 1500 the urban population constituted between 10 and 20 per cent. The Medieval skeletal samples are divided into three categories, central European Early Medieval skeletons, central European Late Medieval skeletons and Scandinavian Medieval skeletons. The central European Early Medieval skeletons were excavated at seven different sites, two in Austria (no reference and Szilvassy 1980), three in Germany (Schnurgein 1987, Neuffer-Müller 1983 and Grünewald 1988) and two in Hungary (Garam 1979 and Nemeskeri 1963). The Scandinavian skeletons originate from six different sites in what was Denmark in the Middle Ages. In fact three of them are situated in Scania which has been a part of Sweden since 1660 (Boldsen 1979 and 1984, Boldsen, Kieffer-Olsen, and Pentz 1985, Persson and Persson 1984, Tkocz and Brøndum 1985 and Mårtensson 1976 and 1981).

All the central European skeletons and most of the Scandinavian skeletons have had their age at death determined by others than the authors. Most of the age categories used can be related to closure of cranial sutures. In the classical German typology three age related anatomical stages have been defined for skeletons of people living to over 18-20 years. These stages comprise **adultus/adulta** (young people with no external closure of the medial sagittal suture), **maturus/matura** (middle aged people with some but not complete closure of the medial sagittal suture) and **senilis/senilia** (older people with complete closure of the medial sagittal suture). No generally accepted ages of transition between these stages exist. In order to give an idea about the range of transition ages it has been estimated in the Danish Medieval Tirup sample that the median maximum-likelihood age estimate at transition from adultus to maturus is 32.5 years and that the standard deviation of this transition is 5.4 years. For the transition from maturus to senilis the corresponding figures are 48.9 and 7.2 years.

Figure 1 illustrates the estimated probabilities of at least having reached the stages adultus/adulta, maturus/matura and senilis/senilia in the Tirup skeletal sample. As expected it appears that the transition into adultus/adulta is much less variable than the transition into maturus/matura and senilis/senilia. This is in accord with the

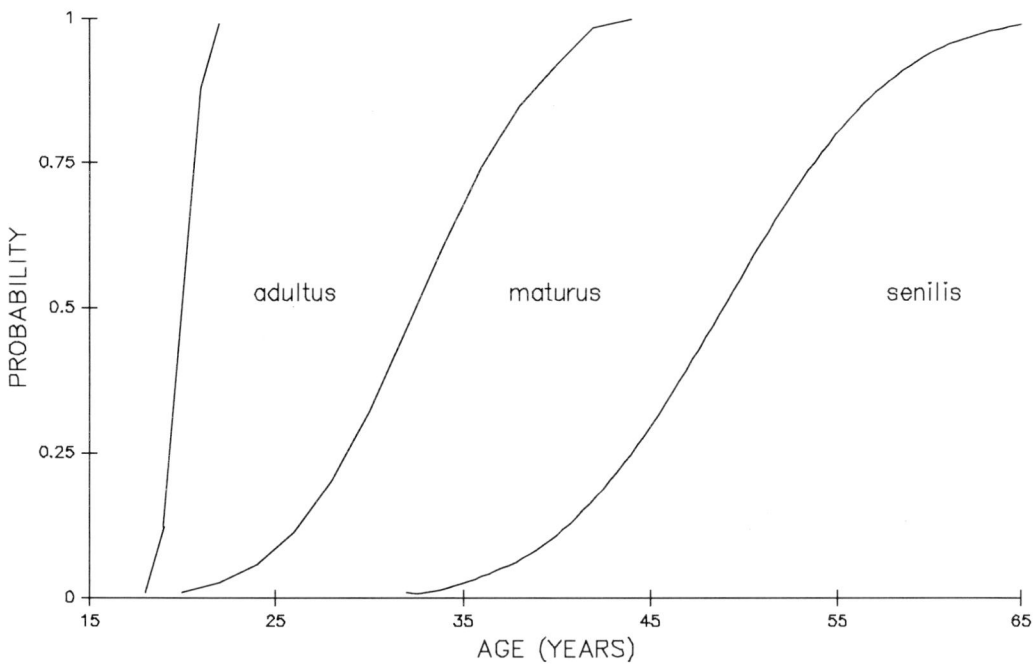

Figure 1: Estimated probabilities of at least having reached each of the age-related anatomical stages 'adultus', 'maturus' and 'senilis'.

general finding that age estimation becomes increasingly inaccurate with increasing age at death. It can be assumed that most females through the studied period only were fertile during adulta.

Results and Discussion

Figure 2 summarizes the development of survival to maturus/matura for the two sexes conditional on survival to around age 18-20.

Females experienced a very serious drop in the probability of reaching matura from the Mesolithic to the subsequent periods. This drop was followed by an increase from Pre-Roman Iron Age and onward. In males nothing seemed to change in the probability of reaching maturus from the Mesolithic to the Pre-Roman Iron Age. The sharp increase in the chance of reaching maturus in males observed in the Roman period is probably a consequence of sample bias. This spike is only based on 191 skeletons from two badly described sites in central Europe.

Cultural evolution was not synchronised in Europe from the Mesolithic to the Middle Ages. Central Europe was usually far in advance of southern Scandinavia. Perhaps Mesolithic foraging was different in coastal Scandinavia and continental central Europe. This might not have had any great demographic consequences; but from the Neolithic revolution the two regions followed different trajectories of cultural evolution dependent on the local environmental conditions, the regional cultural dynamics and impulses received from the rest of the World.

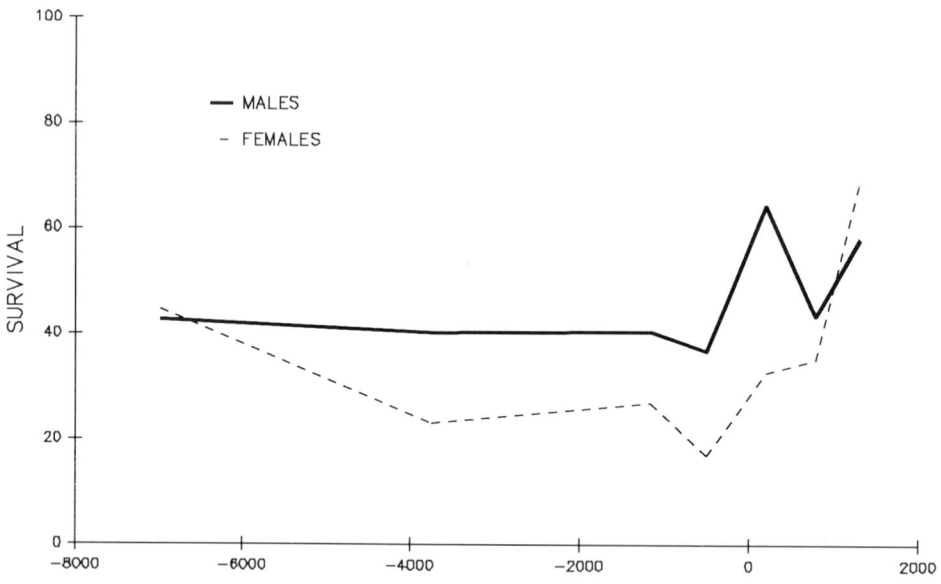

Figure 2: Adult male and female survival (in percent) from age 18-20 to the stage 'maturus/matura' from the Mesolithic to the Medieval period based on central European skeletal samples.

Figure 3 illustrates the development of the chance of reaching maturus/matura in males and females from southern Scandinavia from the Early Roman Iron Age to the Middle Ages. The structure of this development is quite different from the structure of the development in central Europe.

In Scandinavia, it appears that the chance of reaching maturus/matura declined from the Early Roman Iron Age to the Middle Ages. However, this is probably due to sampling bias. The Danish Roman Iron Age skeletal sample is heavily dominated by the upper classes, the regional or national élite of those days. The Medieval samples on the other hand have been selected to represent the general population in various parts of the region. This interpretation is supported by the fact that in all

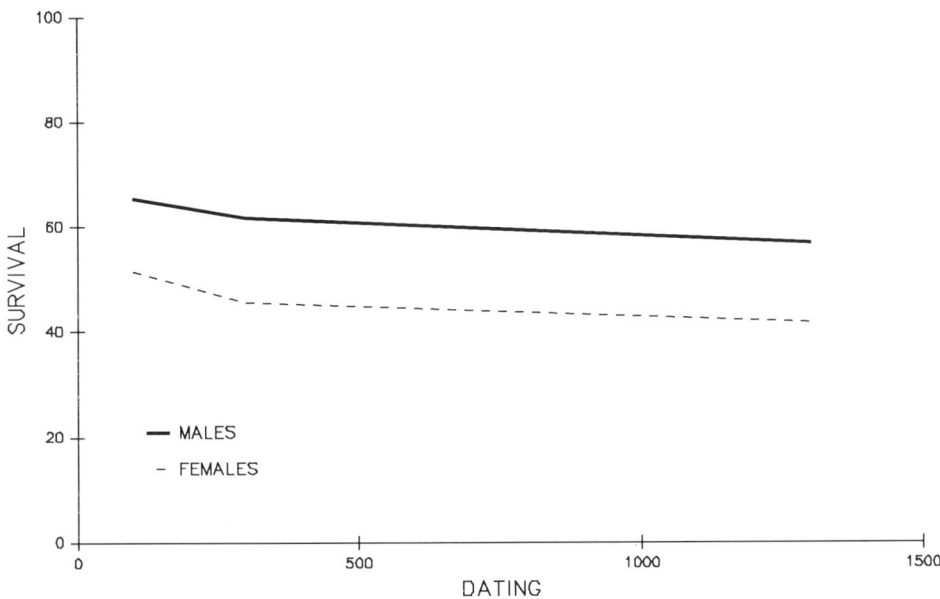

Figure 3: The survival to the stage 'maturus/matura' for males and females from Early Roman Iron Age (AD 0-200), Late Roman Iron Age (AD 200-400) and the Middle Ages (AD 1000-1536) in Denmark.

three periods survivorship is greater in the Scandinavian series than in the central European series.

A preliminary summary conclusion about the evolution of the patterns of adult mortality over the last 8-9000 years is summarized in Figure 4.

Figure 4 is based primarily on the data presented in Figure 2. However, the points for Roman Iron Age and the late Middle Ages have been omitted and the latter have been replaced with much larger and much better described data from southern Scandinavia. As an illustration of the dramatic demographic changes in recent centuries the survivorship to age 40 given survivorship to age 20 is shown for contemporary Denmark. Figure 4 shows a u-shaped curve for the female chance of surviving to matura and a constant curve of the male chance with an increase starting in the Iron Ages. Great differences in the level of survivorship among the sexes persisted well into the second millennium AD.

Three of the four urban samples from Medieval southern Scandinavia show no significant female adult surplus mortality. Only one urban sample (Sct. Mikkel - situated just outside the city wall) shows a significant female surplus mortality. On the other hand, both the two large rural samples do show a highly significant female

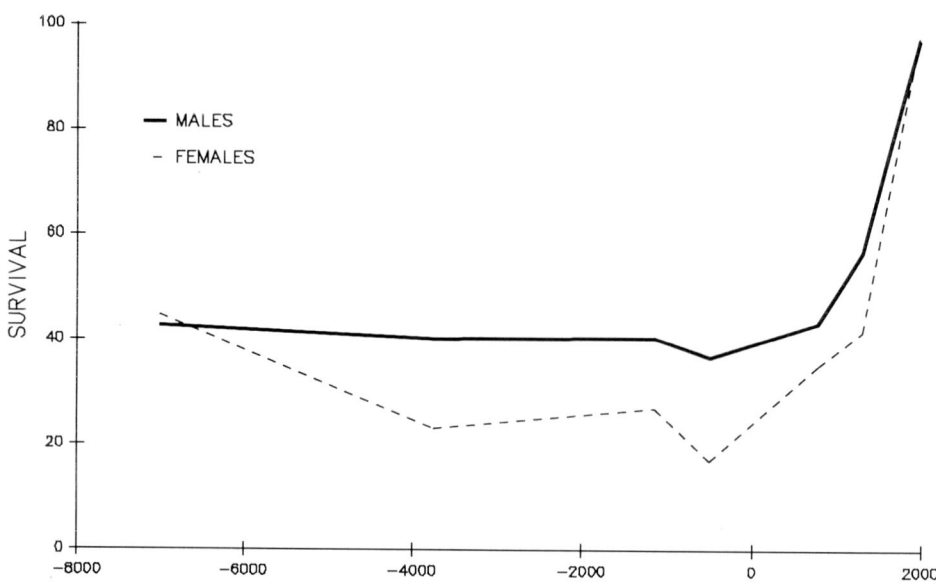

Figure 4: The development of the probability of surviving to 'maturus' for adult males and females from the Mesolithic to the present - a liberal combination of the data shown in figures 2 and 3.

surplus mortality. It is worth noting that the structure of the female adult surplus mortality differs among the urban Sct. Mikkel sample and the rural Löddeköpinge and Tirup samples (Boldsen 1984 and 1988). In the Sct. Mikkel sample the surplus mortality is concentrated among the youngest adult females (ages 18-25 years). In the two rural samples a large fraction of the female surplus mortality is due to deaths among more mature women (ages 30-40 years). The patterns of dental and joint disease in the rural Tirup sample indicate that reproductive depletion among women aged 35-45 years was a common associate of death.

The data presented and analysed in this chapter indicate that adult female surplus mortality is associated with pre-modern agricultural production. It is not possible to determine whether this association is brought about by a heavy work burden, by high fertility or by the microbiological environment of the sedentary, crop-raising communities of Europe from the Neolithic to the late Middle Ages.

In conclusion, it appears that the steady increase of human adult survival - both male and female - is a fairly new phenomenon in hominid evolution. For the males the crude data analysed here indicate a decline in mortality starting in the Early Middle Ages, during or after the fall of the Roman Empire. This late decline of male mortality is paralleled by the females. The decline is even more pronounced among females than among males. The increase of female mortality leading to the decline of survival from the Mesolithic to the Neolithic is probably a very important shift in the selectional forces shaping our species. If this finding can be substantiated by the inclusion of more European data and information from other parts of the world it might provide guidelines for the analysis and understanding of post-glacial demographic evolution.

Literature

Albrethsen, S., and E. Brinch Petersen. 1976. Excavation of a Mesolithic Cemetery at Vedbaek, Denmark. *Acta Archaeologica* 47:1-28.

Bach, A. 1978. Neolithische Population in Mittelelbe-Saale-Gebiet. *Museum für Ur- und Frühgeschichte Thüringens*, Weimar.

Berner, M. (N.D.) Das frühbronzezeitliche Graberfeld von Franzhausen 1, Niederösterreich. Teil 2: Demographische Analyse. *Anthroprologische Abteilung, Naturhistorisches Museum Wien*, Wien.

Bertemes, F. 1989. Das frühbronzezeitliche Graberfeld von Gemeinlebarn. *Saarbrücker Beitrage zur Altertumskunde* 45. Rudolf Habelt GMBH, Bonn.

Boldsen, J.L. 1979. Life and death in Medieval Viborg. Results from the skeletal excavation at the Sct. Mikkels Cemetery (in Danish). *MIV (Museer i Viborg Amt)*, 8:76-85.

Boldsen, J.L. 1984. The Löddeköpinge Investigation IV: Palaeodemography of two Southern Scandinavian Medieval Communities. *Papers of the Archaeological Institute University of Lund 1983-1984.* new series 5:107-115.

Boldsen, J.L. 1988. Two Methods for reconstructing the empirical mortality profile. *Human Evolution* 3:335-342.

Boldsen, J.L., J. Kieffer-Olsen, and P. Pentz. 1985. Således fik kongen bugt med jydernes stivsind. *Skalk* 4:6-10.

Boldsen, J.L., and J. Vellev. 1980. The abandoned Cemetery (Danish). *Skalk* 4:9-15.

Buchvaldik, M., and D. Koutecky. 1970. Vikletice: Ein Schnurkeramisches Graberfeld. *Praehistoria III. Acta Instituti Praehistorici Universitatis Carolinae Pragensis*, Praha.

Czarnetzki, A. 1966. Die menschlichen Skelettreste aus vier neolithischen Steinkisten Hessens und Niedersachsens. *Dissertation Eberhard-Karls-Universität*, Tübingen.

Ehgartner, W. 1959. Die Schadel aus dem frühbronzezeitlichen Graberfeld von Hainburg, Niederosterreich. *Mitteilungen der anthropologischen Gesellschaft in Wien*, 88-89:8-90.

Ehardt, S., and P. Simon. 1971. Skelettfunde der Urnenfelder und Hallstattkultur in Württemberg und Hohenzollern.

Ery, K. 1973. Anthropological Data to the Late Roman Population at Pecs, Hungary. *Anthrop.Hung.* XII:63.

Garam, E. 1979. Das awarenzeitliche Graberfeld von Kirkore. *Akademiai Kiado*, Budapest.

Gejvall, N.G. 1960. Westerhus. Medieval Population and Church in the Light of Skeletal Remains. Lund.

Genesis (Første Mosebog) Bibelen, Den Hellige Skrifts Kanoniske Bøger. *Bibelselskabet for Danmark*, København, 1936:1-60.

Grimm, H. 1958. Die Schnurkeramiker von Schafstadt. *Jahresschrift für Mitteldeutsche Vorgeschichte*, 41, Max Niemeyer, Halle.

Grimm, H. 1959. Weitere Untersuchungen über vorgeschichtliche Menschenreste von Schafstadt. *Jahresschrift für Mitteldeutsche Vorgeschichte*, 43, Max Niemeyer, Halle.

Grimm, H. 1961. Die Schnurkeramiker von Schafstadt. *Jahresschrift für Mitteldeutsche Vorgeschichte*, 45, Max Niemeyer, Halle.

Grünewald, C. 1988. Das alemannische Graberfeld von Unterthurheim, Bayerysche-Schwaben. *M. Lassleben*, Kallmünz.

Jensen, J. 1988. Gyldendal og Politikens Danmarkshistorie. Bind 1: I begyndelsen - Fra de ældste tider til ca. år 200 f.Kr. *Gyldendalske Boghandel and Politikens Forlag*, Copenhagen.

Kramer, W. 1964. Das keltische Graberfeld von Nebringen (Kreis Boblingen). *Verlag Silberburg*, Stuttgart.

Kreiling, H. 1979. Glovzin: Ein Urnenfriedhof der vorrömerischen Eisenzeit im Kreis Perleberg. *VEB Deutscher Verlag der Wissenschaften*, Berlin.

Larsson, L. 1989. The Skateholm Project I. Man and Environment. *Almqvist & Wiksell International*, Stockholm.

Mallory, J.P. 1989. In Search of the Indo-Europeans. Language, Archaeology and Myth. *Thames and Hudson Ltd*, London.

Mårtensson, A.W. 1976. Uppgrävt förflutet för PKbanken i Lund. *Kulturhistoriska Museet i Lund*, Malmö.

Mårtensson, A.W. 1981. S:t Stefans Lund. Ett monument ur tiden. *Gamla Lund, Förening för bevarende av stadens minnen Årsskrift* 62, Lund.

Nemeskeri, J. 1963. Die spätmittelalterliche Bevolkerung von Fonyod. *Anthropologia Hungarica*, 6:87-115.

Neuffer-Müller, C. 1983. Der alemannische Adelbestattungsplatz und die Reihengraberfriedhöfe von Kirchheim am Reis. Forschungen und Berichte zur Vor- und Frühgeschichte in Baden Württemberg. Bd 15, *K. Theiss Verlag*, Stuttgart.

Patte, E. 1971. Les Restes Humains de la Grotte Sepulcrale du Laris Goguet a Feigneux (Oise). *Bulletins et Menoires de la Societe d'Anthropologie de Paris*, 7:381-452.

Persson, P.O., and E. Persson. 1983. The Löddeköpinge Investigation V. Report on the anthropometrics of the skeletons from the early medieval cemetery in

Löddeköpinge (Scania, S. Sweden). *University of Lund Institute of Archaeology, Report Series No. 19*.

Rasmussen, L.W. 1990. Dolkproduktion og -distribution i senneolitikum. *Hikuin* 16:31-42.

Saller, K. 1962. Die Ofnet: Funde in neuer Zusammenseitung. Ihre Stellung in der Rassengeschichte Europas. *Zeitschrift der Morphologie und Anthropologie* 57:1-51.

Sawyer, P. 1988. Gyldendal og Politikens Danmarkshistorie. Bind 3: Da Danmark blev Danmark. Fra ca. år 700 til ca. 1050. *Gyldendalske Boghandel and Politikens Forlag*, Copenhagen.

Schnurgein, A. 1987. Der alemannische Friedhof bei Fridingen an der Donau (Kreis Tuttlingen). *K. Theiss*, Stuttgart.

Schwidetzky, I. 1978. Anthropologie der Dürnberger Bevolkerung. In Pauli, L (ed) Der Dürnnberg bei Hallein III. *C.S. Beck*, München.

Sellevold, B.J., U.L. Hansen, and J.B. Jørgensen. 1984. Iron Age Man in Denmark, Prehistoric Man in Denmark vol 3. *Det Kongelige Nordiske Oldskriftselskab*, Copenhagen.

Spindler, K. 1977. Der Hallstattzeitliche Fürstengrabhügen bei Villingen im Schwarzwald. *Magdalenenberg* 5.

Szilvassy, J. 1980. Die Skelette aus dem awarischen Graberfeld von Zwolfaxing in Niederösterreich. *Ferdinand Berger & Sohne*, Wien.

Tkocz, I., and N. Brøndum. 1985. Anthropological Analyses. Medieval Skeletons from the Franciscan Cemetery in Svendborg. *The Archaeology of Svendborg, Denmark, No. 3. Odense University Press*, Odense.

Patterns of Advanced Age Mortality in the Medieval Village Tirup

by Jesper L. Boldsen

The general Medieval rural Danish population rarely entered contemporary written records. These people formed the basis of most of the events which took place, but they have left pitifully few individual marks. The drama of the life of the individual Medieval peasant escapes our comprehension. The marks of their lives and labour can be seen in the Romanesque churches scattered throughout the country and in the names of their settlements. However, the only direct source of knowledge about the individual man, woman and child in the Middle Ages are the skeletons of the people themselves. The unique historical character of each individual life story is generated in a confrontation between the general period and group specific conditions of living and the actual course of events that formed life. Some life history events like birth and death have general importance more or less independent of time and place. But in spite of this, the perception of such events is strongly dependent on ideological fabric creating meaning in the life of the individual in the present as well as in the past and on the less elusive conditions of living and producing.

The demography of the Medieval Danish population is one of the few areas where it is presently possible to approach a thorough description of one objective side of the frame of living in the past. Benedictow (1993) has given an overview over some general trends in the demography of Medieval communities in Scandinavia. Part of this work builds on case studies of osteodemography and population structure of the individual finds (Boldsen 1979 and 1984, Brøste 1945, Gejvall 1960, Holk 1970 and 1987, Högberg et al. 1987, Møller-Christensen 1953, Persson and Persson 1981, Persson 1976, Siven 1991a and 1991b, Sjøvold 1978 and Tkocz 1985). In spite of the fairly large number of case studies of Scandinavian Medieval demography only three totally excavated rural parish cemeteries from the Nordic area have been published, Westerhus in Sweden (Gejvall 1960), Thjorhilde's Church in Greenland (Lynnerup 1995) and Tirup in Denmark (Kieffer-Olsen, Boldsen and Pentz 1986).

The validity of results from palaeodemographic research has been seriously questioned both locally (eg Olsen 1982) and in the general biological anthropological literature (eg Bocquet-Appel and Masset 1982). The controversy following some of this criticism has led to the appearance of papers pointing to other problems of the application of quantitative osteological methods in the study of growth- and health-related processes in past communities (Wood, Milner, Harpending and Weiss 1992 and Saunders and Hoppa 1993). Work is in progress trying to solve some of the problems pointed to by Wood et al. (1992) and Saunders and Hoppa (1993) and utilizing Scandinavian skeletal samples for this end. The purpose of the present chapter is to analyse aspects of the pattern of adult mortality in the Early Medieval Tirup community in eastern Jutland, Denmark, with the aim of gleaning information on the probability of surviving to advanced ages.

Material and methods

The Tirup cemetery was in use from around AD 1100 to after 1300 (Kieffer-Olsen 1993). Only a small part of the area possibly containing the remains of the village to which the church and the cemetery belonged has been investigated. However, the lack of reference to the site in late Medieval written sources indicate that the place and community lost its independent importance by the middle of the 14th century. The name of the community, Tirup, gives a clue to the foundation of the village. The -rup ending of the name indicates a -torp type of village. The -torp type villages were founded in the Viking Age and during the early Middle Ages by moving existing farms and establishing new ones in areas marginal to older villages. The majority of these -torp villages were probably founded in the 11th and 12th century AD (Sawyer 1988). This means that it is likely that the excavated cemetery spans the whole history of the Tirup community. The area which came to form the cemetery had not been in profane use during the Viking age and the earliest parts of the Middle Ages. Judging from the ceramics and structures found under the cemetery the area had not been in regular use since the Bronze Age (Kieffer-Olsen, Boldsen and Pentz 1986). These circumstances indicate that the skeletons found in the Tirup cemetery are unique in representing the total population of a small village (on average some 70 inhabitants - cf. Boldsen 1994) throughout its whole existence of some 200 years.

The Tirup cemetery was excavated in 1984. The area used for burials was surrounded by a well-defined ditch. The whole area within the ditch and a strip of 5-10 meters outside of it was excavated. No graves were found outside the circumscribed area. Evidence of 618 burials were found (Kieffer-Olsen, Boldsen and Pentz 1986). It is assumed that around 100 infant burials were not recovered due to the grave not penetrating beneath the top soil (Boldsen, Kieffer-Olsen and Pentz, work in progress). This chapter is only concerned with adult mortality. This means that the absence of some infant burials in the material does not affect the results. The material for the present analyses consists of 116 male and 95 female skeletons from Tirup.

The material analysed here consists of skeletons in which it has been possible to determine age at death and sex. The indicators of sex are very vague for individuals younger than 18-20 years at death. This means that only skeletons clearly indicating an age above 18 years are included in the analyses. The methods of the determination of sex and of age at death are described by Boldsen (1988). The empirical mortality profiles have been reconstructed from the two sets of age at death intervals (male and female) using a method first described by Turnbull (1978) and developed for the reconstruction of palaeodemographic profiles by Boldsen (1984 and 1988). This method treats the skeletal data as interval censored data. The method gives unbiased estimates of the distribution of age at death but it does not facilitate rigorous statistical testing.

Under the stationary population model the cumulative distribution of age at death corresponds to one minus the survival function. Mortality rates estimated from the mortality profiles estimated in this way are virtually independent of natural population growth or decline; but they are vulnerable to age and sex specific migration. The Tirup community is assumed to have gone through an initial phase of natural immigration mediated population growth followed possibly after a period of fluctuating population size by a depopulation phase. Nothing indicates that the community went extinct in a demographic catastrophe (Boldsen, Kieffer-Olsen and Pentz, work in progress). The Tirup community was probably one of the rural communities that supplied the young adult immigrants found in some Medieval urban cemeteries like Sct. Mikkel in Viborg some 80 km north of Tirup (cf. Boldsen 1984). It has been estimated that as much as 40% of adult females buried in this cemetery were immigrants from surrounding rural communities like Tirup. However, the Medieval urban communities contained a maximum of 10% of the population and the migrants consisted of women under the age of 22 years. As the estimates of the mortality rates are independent of events (death and/or migration) taking place prior to the age under study this means that emigration from the community had a negligible effect on the mortality rates estimated from the mortality profiles.

The endpoints of the age intervals forming the data for the analyses in this chapter show a clear digit preference. The vast majority of endpoints (both upper and lower) have a last digit of '0' or '5'. To correct for the bias introduced by this digit preference the mortality profiles have been smoothed out in the way described by Boldsen (1988). The yearly mortality rates estimated directly from mortality profiles are quite unstable even after having smoothed the profiles. In order to make the mortality rates more stable they have been estimated as ten year moving averages as follows:

$$\mu(t) = - \ln \{ M(t+5) / M(t-5) \} / 10,$$

where '$\mu(t)$' is the mortality rate at age 't', '$M(t)$' is the value of the smoothed mortality profile at age 't' and 'ln' is the natural (base e) logarithm. For comparison the mortality rates of the contemporary Danish populations (1990-91) have been estimated in the same way just using the survival function rather than the mortality profile as the basis for the calculations (Statistisk Årbog 1993).

Results and discussion

The basic differences in the mortality patterns among the peasants from Tirup and recent Danes are clearly illustrated in Figure 1.

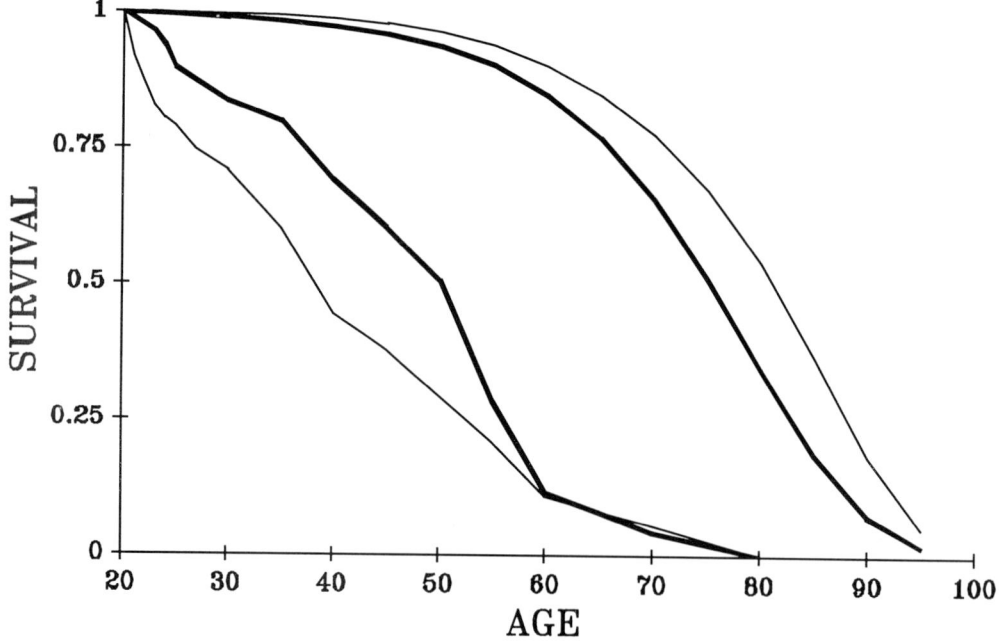

Figure 1 The mortality profile/survival function for the Tirup cemetery (lower curves) and recent Danes (upper curves). Heavy lines: males, light lines: females.

This figure illustrates the empirical mortality profile for the Tirup cemetery conditioned on age at death over 20 years and the survival function conditional on survival to age 20 years for recent Danes. It is well-known that survival is higher for both sexes and at all ages for the recent Danes than is was for the people of Tirup. It has also been shown before that early adult survival was greater in males than in females in Tirup. The fact that the Tirup mortality profiles are based on relatively few observations is illustrated by the generally unsmooth curves that these functions draw.

The curves in Figure 1 have been translated to the mortality rates illustrated on a logarithmic scale in Figure 2.

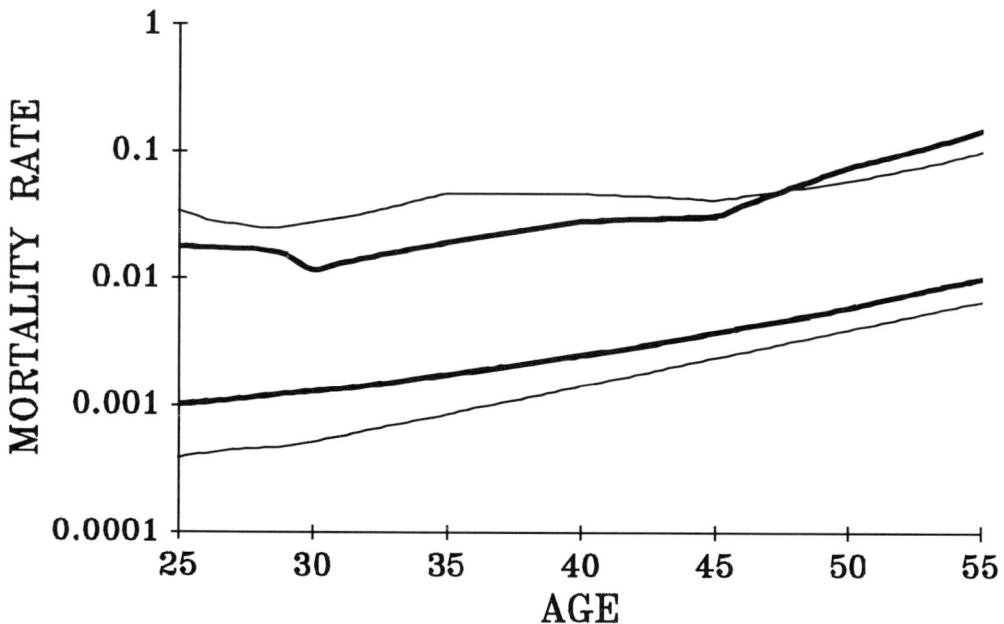

Figure 2 Mortality rates for the Tirup (upper curves) and for the recent Danes (lower curves). Females: light curves males: heavy curves.

This figure illustrates the general similarity and the great difference between the patterns of mortality in the Tirup community and in Denmark today. All four curves in Figure 2 show evidence of an increase of the mortality rate from young adulthood (20-30 years) to later adulthood (50-60 years). In contemporary Denmark this development is monotonous whereas in Tirup the youngest adults (ages around 25 years) experienced a higher mortality rate than did people in their early thirties. This is just a minor difference between the two sets of mortality rates. The most striking difference is that the mortality rates in Tirup were never less than five times as high as the mortality rates for the same sex and age in contemporary Denmark.

The surplus mortality in the Tirup community is illustrated in Figure 3. It appears that female surplus mortality in Tirup was larger than male surplus mortality in all ages from 25 to 55 years; but the curves converge from age 40 and onward reaching very similar levels at 55 (mortality rate ratio of 8.9 for females versus 7.6 for males). The determination of age at death is at best very inaccurate and the number of skeletons available for study is small for ages over 50 years in all pre-modern societies. The general flat curve for the male mortality rate ratio for ages over 35 years and the converges of the male and female curves at the upper end of the age spectrum illustrated in Figure 3 indicates that it might be fruitful to study old age mortality in a community like Tirup by multiplying the mortality rates for recent Danes by a constant.

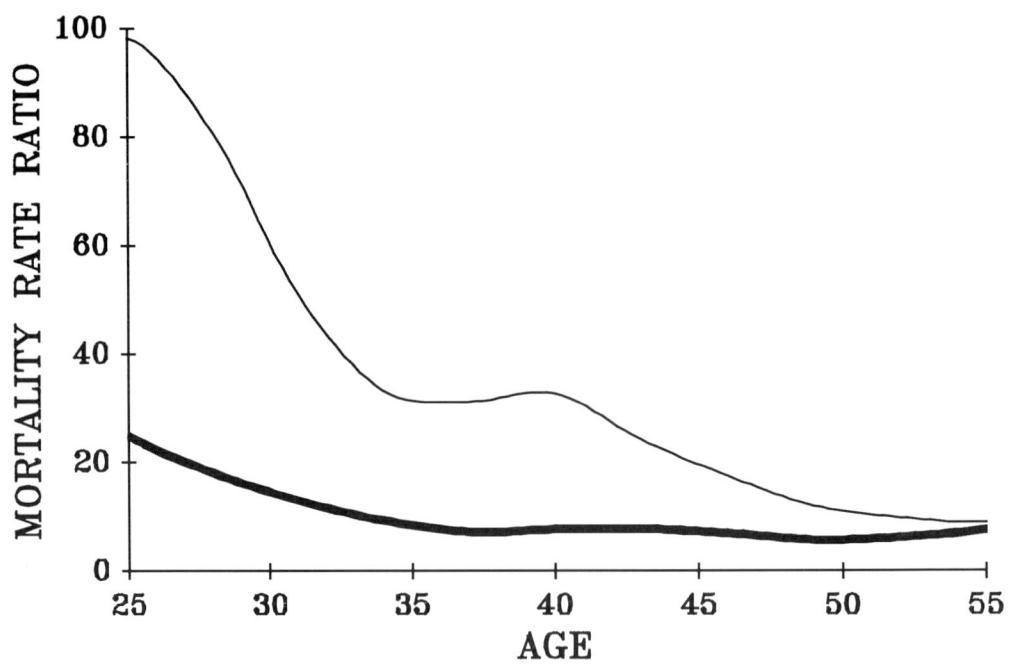

Figure 3 Mortality rate ratio (Tirup versus contemporary Danes) for males (heavy curve) and females (light curve) for ages from 25 - 55 years.

Following this reasoning Figure 4 probably illustrates the best possible reconstruction of the survival function for a Medieval village community in Denmark conditioned on survival to age 50 years. It might be a point of interest that using the mortality rate ratio factor 8 the chance of surviving to age 100 was $3.8*10^{-19}$ for males and $7.1*10^{-16}$ for females given that the person had lived to reach age 50 (see Vaupel and Jeune, in this monograph, for discussion of this calculation). Less than 25 percent of the males and 15 percent of the females in Tirup reached age 50. The mean survival time at age 50 is 25.6 years for males and 29.9 years for females in contemporary Denmark. Following the same method used to reach the figures behind Figure 4 it can be calculated that the mean survival time in the Tirup community at age 50 was 9.8 and 12.6 years for males and females, respectively.

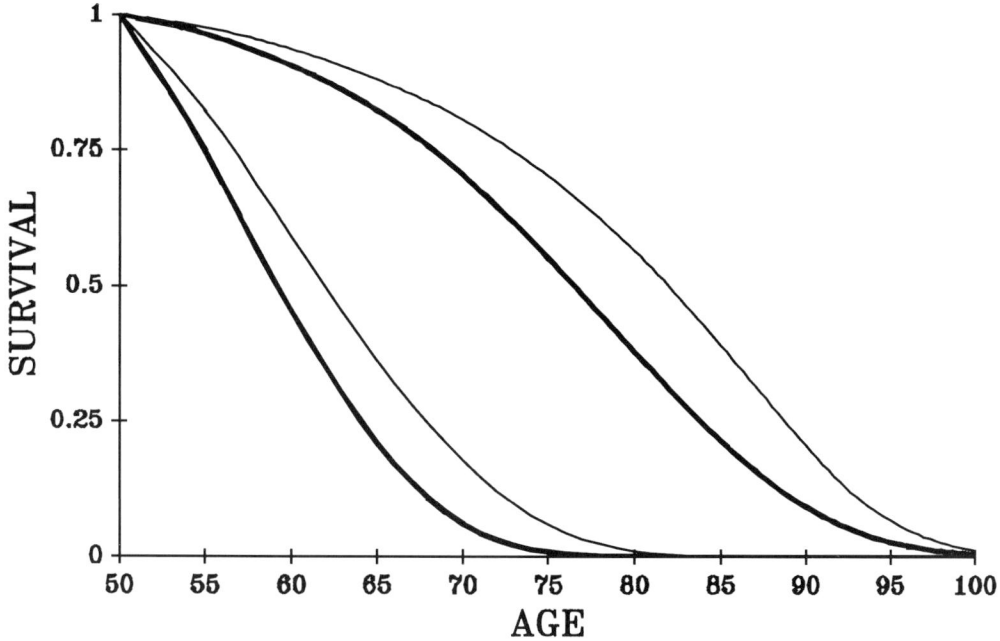

Figure 4 Survival functions from age 50 years reconstructed for the Tirup community (lower curves) and calculated for recent Danes (upper curves). Heavy curves: males, light curves: females.

The Tirup village probably experiences some 700 births through its whole history. This means that an expected 34 males and 25 females would have reached the age of 60 years before dying. Of these 5 men and 8 women are expected to have reached the age of 70 years. The expected number of both men and women reaching the age of 80 years is less than one (0.03 males and 0.4 females). A reasonable estimate of the number of people born to the rural Danish population through the Middle Ages is close to 20,000,000 (based on a crude mortality rate of 0.05 and an average population of between 500,000 and 1,000,000 people in a 500 year period). Of these in excess of 1/4 of a million would have reached the age of 70 years, around 12,000 would have reached 80 and only four of them (all females) are expected to have reached the age of 90 years. The estimated number of persons reaching the really high age of 100 years is $8.8*10^{-10}$. This means that the chance for any member of the rural Medieval Danish community or of any community with a similar pattern of mortality of living a full century is effectively nil.

Wilmoth (in this monograph) has given a very strict definition of the emergence of the first centenarians. He requires a 99% probability of at least one centenarian appearing in the world population each century. This corresponds to a mean number of centenarians each century of close to five (4.6). Following this criterion a world population with the pattern of mortality seen in the Medieval Danish village of Tirup should consist of more than 10^{17} people. This many people have never existed and it must be concluded that the Tirup mortality regime would never have produced even a single centenarian. The difference between this conclusion and the conclusion reached by Wilmoth (in this monograph) is probably not a consequence of the empirical data used for the estimation of the chance to reach 100 years. Both approaches vastly extrapolate any results that could be reached on empirical grounds. This extrapolation is most serious for the oldest age mortality, i.e. mortality from 90 to 100 years of age. This means that although the present analysis reaches a conclusion incompatible with the one reached by Wilmoth (in this monograph), the differences are solely due to differences in assumptions, and I for one would not insist that my own more empirical approach gives more reliable results than the more model-orientated approach used by Wilmoth. Further, the analyses indicate that the solution to the contradiction lies in the acquisition and analysis of more and more reliable data on mortality in antiquity.

Literature

Benedictow, O.J. 1993. The Medieval Demographic System of the Nordic Countries. *Middelalderforlaget*, Oslo.

Bocquet-Appel, J.P., and C. Masset. 1982. Farewell to Paleodemography. *Journal of Human Evolution* 11:321-334.

Boldsen, J.L. 1979. Life and Death in Medieval Viborg. Results from the excavation of skeletons on Sct. Mikkels Kirkegård (in Danish). *MIV (Museer i Viborg Amt)* 8:76-85.

Boldsen, J.L. 1984. The Löddeköpinge investigation IV: Palaeodemography of two southern Scandinavian Medieval communities. *Papers form the Archaeological Institute, University of Lund, new series* 5:105-115.

Boldsen, J.L. 1988. Two methods for the reconstruction of the empirical mortality profile. *Human Evolution* 3:335-342.

Boldsen, J.L. 1994. Migration and community size in early Medieval Jutland - a simulation study. In Marker, H.J., and K. Pagh (ed) Yesterday - proceedings from the 6th international conference Association of History and Computing, Odense 1991, 182-91. *Odense University Press*, Odense.

Brøste, K. 1945. The find of skeletons in the Medieval round building in Malling (in Danish). *Aarbøger for Nordisk Oldkyndighed og Historie* 1945, 156-166.

Gejvall, N.G. 1960. Westerhus, Medieval Population and Church in the Light of Skeletal Remains. Lund.

Holk, P. 1970. Ein Bericht über die Untersuchung der ausgegrabenen Skelette aus der Kirsche aus Mære. *Skrifter utgitt av Det Norske Videnskabs-Akademi i Oslo. Mat.-Naturv. Klasse, New Series*, No. 28:1-66.

Holk, P. 1987. The skeletal material from Peterskirken, Tønsberg. An anthropological report (in Norwegian). *Antropologiske Skrifter, No. 2*, Department of Anatomy, University of Oslo.

Kieffer-Olsen, J. 1993. Grave and burial custom in Medieval Denmark - 8 cemetery excavations (in Danish). Ph.D thesis, *Department of Medieval Archaeology*, Moesgaard, Århus.

Kieffer-Olsen, J., J.L. Boldsen, and P. Pentz. 1986. A newly found church at Bygholm (in Danish). *Vejle Amts Årbog 1986* 24-51.

Lassen, A. 1965. Decline and Rise - aspects of population development in Denmark 1645-1960 (in Danish). *Universitetsforlaget*, København.

Lynnerup, N. 1994. The Greenland Norse - a biological anthropological study. Unpublished thesis, University of Copenhagen.

Olsen, O. 1982. The quantitative approach in urban archaeology. *C.B.A. Research Report* 43: 6-9.

Saunders, S.R., and R.D. Hoppa. 1993. Growth deficit in survivors and non-survivors: Biological Mortality Bias in Subadult Skeletal Samples. *Yearbook of Physical Anthropology* 36: 127-151.

Sawyer, P. 1988. When Denmark became Denmark. From ca. 700 to ca. 1050 (in Danish). *Gyldendal og Politikens Danmarkshistorie bind 3*, København.

Siven, C.H. 1991. On estimating Mortality from Osteological Age Data. *International Journal of Anthropology* 6: 97-110.

Siven, C.H. 1991. On reconstructing the (once) Living Population from Osteological Data. *International Journal of Anthropology* 6: 111-118.

Sjøvold, T. 1978. Skeletal finds (in Swedish). in *One Thousand years on the Church Spit. Leksand Church, archaeology and Building history* 165-170.

Statistisk Årbog. 1993. (Statistical Yearbook), *Danmarks Statistik*, Copenhagen.

Tkocz, I. 1985. Skeletal Material from the Layman's Churchyard. in *The Archaeology of Svendborg* 26-63.

Turnbull, B.W. 1976. The empirical distribution function with arbitrarily grouped, censored and truncated data. *Journal Royal Statistical Society B* 38: 290-295.

Vaupel, J.W., and B. Jeune. 1994. The Emergence and Proliferation of Centenarians. *Population Studies of Ageing #12*, Centre for Health and Social Policy, Odense University, Denmark.

Wilmoth, J.R. 1995. The Earliest Centenarians: A Statistical Analysis. (in this monograph).

Wood, J.W., G.R. Milner, H.C. Harpending, and K.M. Weiss. 1992. The Osteological Paradox: Problems of inferring prehistoric health from skeletal samples. *Current Anthropology* 33: 343-370.

Alleged Danish Centenarians before 1800

by Thorkild Kjærgaard

The first Dane known to have studied old age was Bolle Willum Luxdorph (1716-88) (Fig.1). He was a high-ranking civil servant in the Danish-Norwegian monarchy, leader of the Danish Chancellery. Luxdorph was a man of wide and varied interests. He cultivated roses, he was well-trained in classical studies and wrote, as one of the last in Denmark, a beautiful Latin. He published poems in Danish and of course in Latin and was a prolific writer in many fields. He was a great book-collector, and he kept a diary every day for decades. This voluminous diary has been published in our century and is one of the most rewarding sources of 18th century Danish-Norwegian history.

Bolle Willum Luxdorph followed various tracks in his studies of old age. He compiled two catalogues of *longævi* ('longlivers'), ie people who had lived 80 years or more, 80 years being from Roman times the beginning of senectitute. He collected pictures of longævi. Finally in 1780 he made an investigation of the phenomenon of centenarians in the Danish-Norwegian monarchy of the late 18th century.

Luxdorph's picture gallery

The first of Luxdorph's two catalogues, both in Latin, was <u>Catalogus longævorum</u> from 1780. This catalogue was never printed, but survives as a beautiful manuscript in the Royal Library of Copenhagen. The second <u>Index tabularurum pictarum et cælatarum qvæ Longævos repræsentant</u> was published in October 1783 on the occasion of the 80th anniversary of Luxdorph's political chief, Count Otto Thott, who is the youngest person mentioned in the catalogue.

Catalogues of longævi were not unknown in the 18th century (see Jeune's introduction to this monograph), eg the Swiss scholar Albrect von Haller had published one in 1760 and earlier in the century a couple of such catalogues had been published in Paris. The extraordinary thing about Luxdorph's catalogues is that he combines his listing of longævi with pictures of the persons in question. The <u>Catalogus longævorum</u>, which incidentally lists 33 centenarians from classical times until 17th century Denmark including a couple of Danish kings, is illustrated with many drawings. The second catalogue from 1783 is, as the title indicates, a catalogue of pictures of longævi, including 36 pictures representing people who claimed to have reached the age of hundred years or more. Altogether the 1783-catalogue lists close to 300 pictures of longævi.

In the following years Luxdorph continued to collect pictures of longævi, and when he died in 1788, at the age of 72, he left a collection of 728 pictures - drawings and prints - of longævi, arranged according to their age, the oldest first and the youngest, those of 80 years, including a few persons still living, last. None of the centenarians, of whom there were now 42, were verified or confirmed. Some of them were well-known European longævi, eg Cathrine of Desmonde (1464-1604). Most of these non-Danish-Norwegian longævi, perhaps all of them, have been refuted in the literature, beginning with the famous studies of Thoms (see Jeune's introduction).

As far as the Danish centenarians or supercentenarians in the Luxdorph picture gallery are concerned they are all impossible to substantiate. Many of them were born abroad, which makes it next to impossible to verify their age claims. That is true of the soldier Anton Crolekofsky, who claimed to be 113 years old when he died in Copenhagen in 1785, and of whom a drawing was made for Luxdorph's gallery by a well-known Copenhagen artist Georg Fuchs (Fig.2). Crolekofsky claimed to have been born in Poland. Abramham Clod de Meer who died 1785, allegedly at the age of 102, was also born abroad. Abraham Clod de Meer, who is supposed to have been the first tobacco planter in Denmark, was reported to have been born in Holland.

The sailor Christian Drakenberg, who towards the end of his life made a living out of being old, claimed to be 146 years old when he died in 1772. He was born in Norway before church registers were common. Drakenberg's totally unsubstantiated claim to high age was unusually inflated and fanciful, but also unusually successful. He was one of the most frequently pictured persons from the non-ruling classes in the 18th century Danish-Norwegian monarchy (Fig.3).

Another centenarian in Luxdorph's gallery is the carpenter Jens Larsen Møller, who died in 1788, allegedly 102 years old, but with no evidence to confirm this (Fig.4). The same goes for the mint-master to Frederik II from the 16th century, and - to put it briefly - for all the rest of the centenarians in the Luxdorph gallery.

Nevertheless, Luxdorph's series of portraits of longævi is highly interesting, probably one of the most unusual collections ever to have existed in Denmark, and certainly one of the most extraordinary Danish contributions to gerontology. Unfortunately the collection was split up and sold together with Luxdorph's other possessions at an auction in 1789. Since then these hundreds of drawings and prints have drifted around, until some of them ended up in museums, including the

Frederiksborg Museum. A reconstruction of Luxdorph's collection in the form of a book has been under consideration for some time and is now under preparation. Hopefully it will be an entertaining as well as a rewarding contribution to the history of gerontology.

The 1780 investigation by Luxdorph

In 1780 Luxdorph wrote to the bishops and a few other high-ranking men of the church in Denmark and Norway, asking them to provide information about the centenarians in their districts - especially those recently deceased. Luxdorph also requested detailed biographies of the alleged centenarians and descriptions of their health. He wanted facts, not fairy-tales, and the clergy were asked to check all information on age with the church registers of baptisms and burials, the registers which had been introduced by law in Denmark in 1645-46 and in Norway in 1685. Apparently not all the clergy responded, but many did, most of them by asking the vicars of the various parishes to provide the answers. The answers were returned to Luxdorph, who collected them, together with some miscellaneous material on old age in a volume of documents called Longævi, today kept at the Royal Library in Copenhagen.

When you study the replies from the Danish and Norwegian clergy you cannot help noticing a significant difference between the material provided by the Danish clergy and that provided by their Norwegian colleagues. The Norwegian clergy mention almost 30 centenarians, while the Danish quote less than 10, although there were more people living in Denmark than in Norway.

There is probably a very simple explanation for this: age exaggeration was relatively easy in Norway, where church registers were introduced nation-wide as late as in 1685, while they were introduced already in 1645-46 in Denmark. This means that in 1780, when Luxdorph was requesting information on centenarians, church registers had only existed nation-wide in Norway for 95 years, except for the relatively few places where church registers had been in use on a voluntary basis before 1680. The parsons in Norway knew of course that people tended to exaggerate their age, but they could not do very much about it apart from adding: he or she claims to have attained this and that age, and that is supported by this and that fact and by his children and all the family, but unfortunately there is no church register to confirm his or her claim.

In Denmark where church registers had existed on a nation-wide basis since the

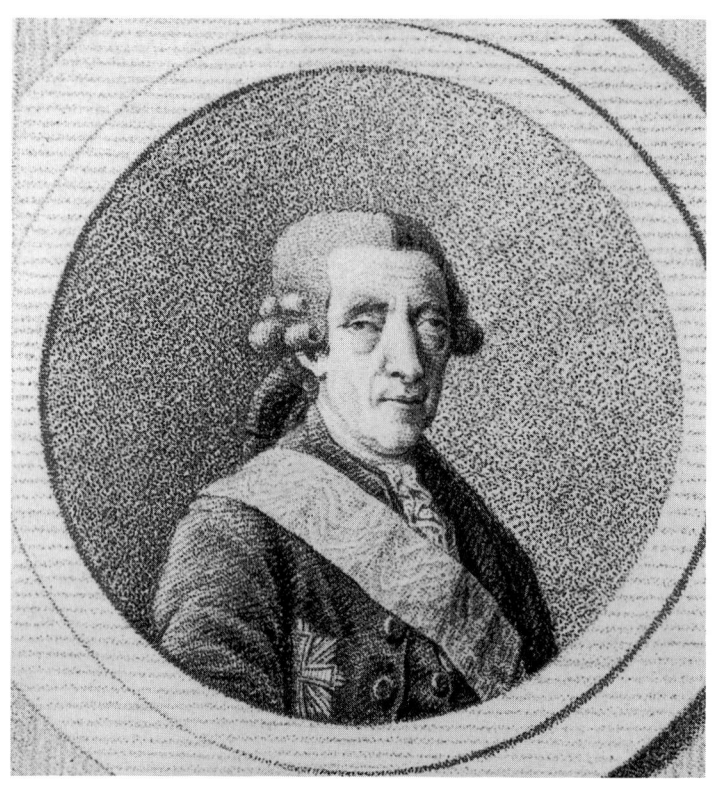

Fig. 1
Bolle Willum Luxdorph (1716-1788). Engraving by T. Kleve, 1781. Frederiksborg Museum, Hillerød.

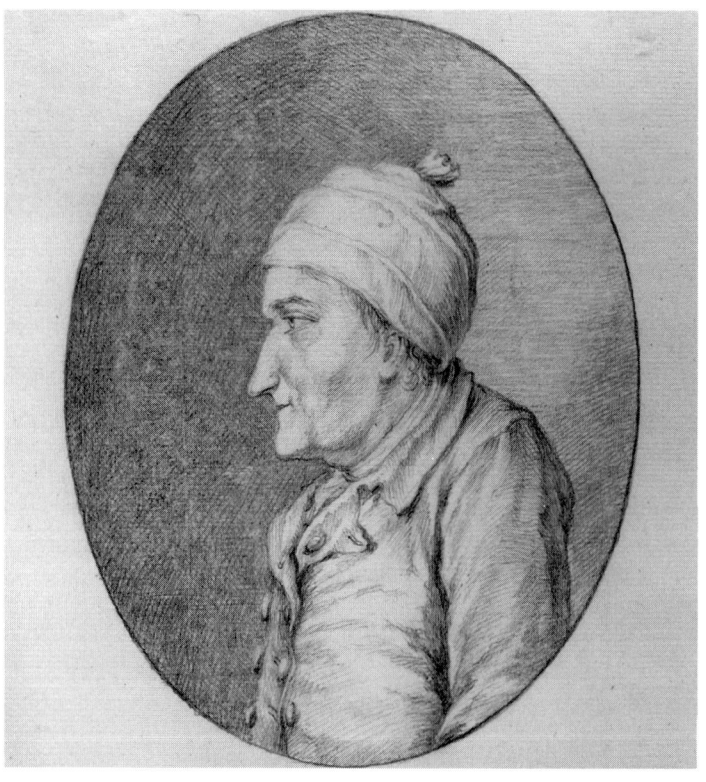

Fig. 2
Anton Crolekofsky (Carolicopsky) (1672?-1785). Drawing by G. Fuchs, 1780. Statens Museum for Kunst, Copenhagen.

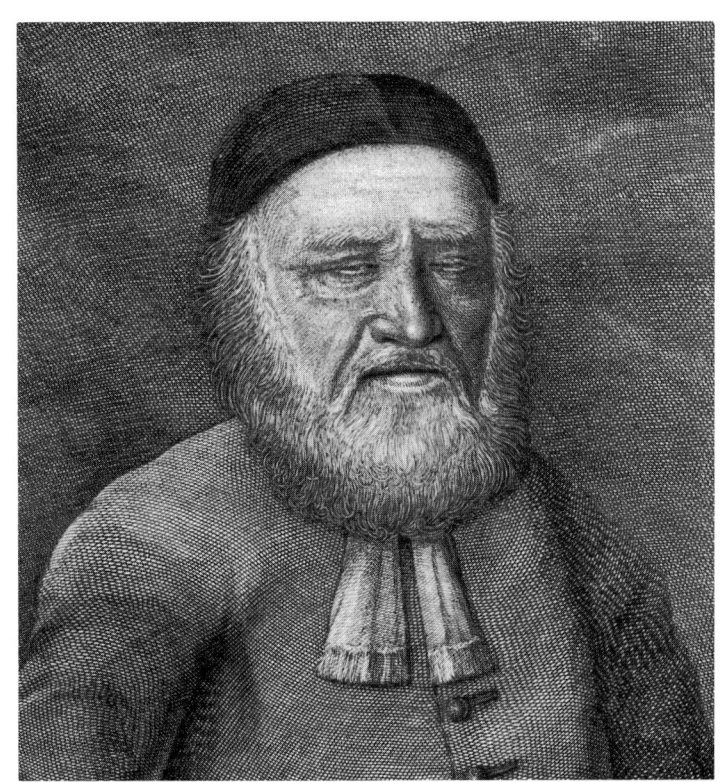

Fig. 3
Christian Drakenberg (1626?-1772). Engraving by C. Fritsch, 1768. Frederiksborg Museum, Hillerød.

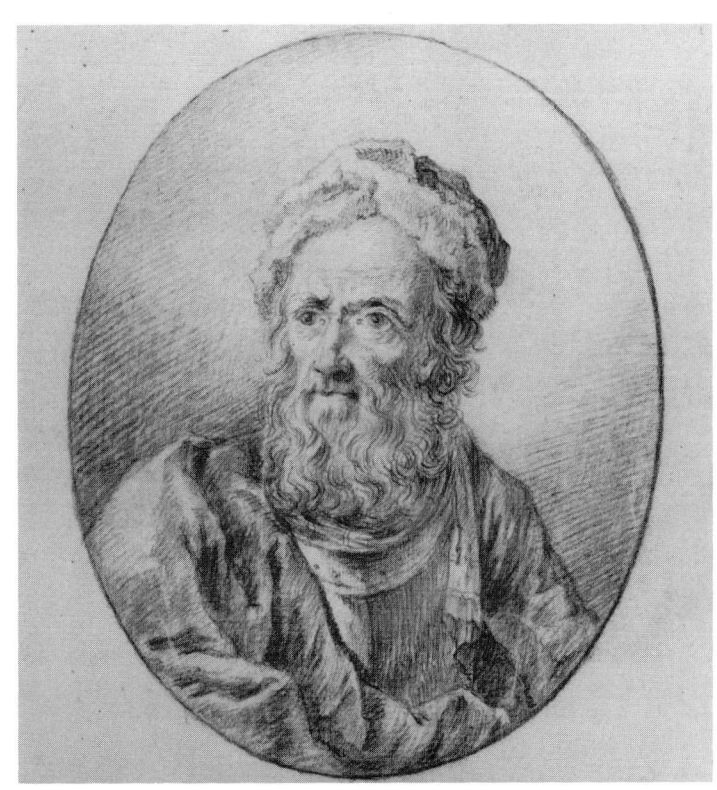

Fig. 4
Jens Larsen Møller (1686?-1788). Drawing by G. Fuchs, 1788. Statens Museum for Kunst, Copenhagen.

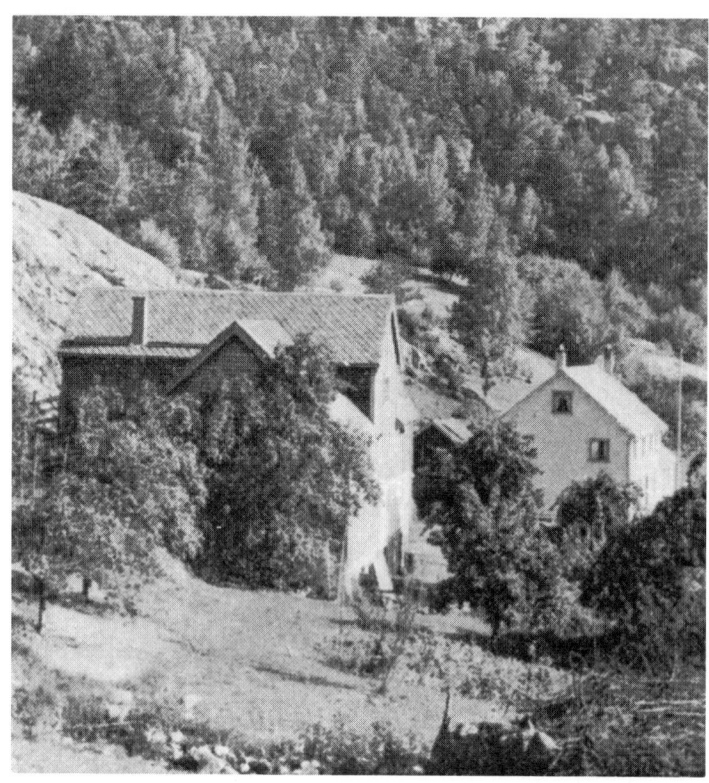

Fig. 5
No picture of Eilif Philipsen exists. Here the farm outside Bergen in Norway, where the first documented centenarian spent his whole life.

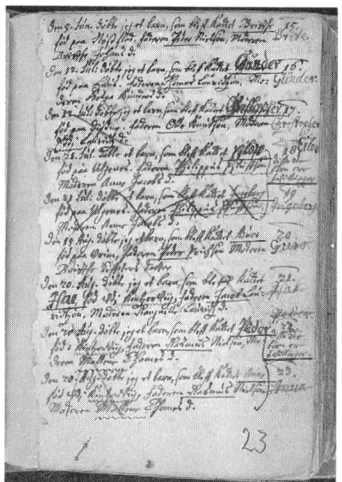 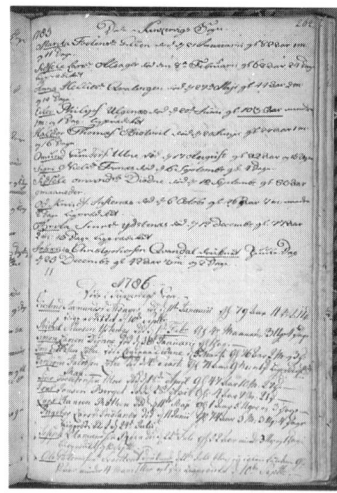

Fig. 6
Two pages from the church register at Kinsarvik. The page on the left from 1682 mentions that the twins Eilif and Ingeborg were christened on 21 July 1682. The page on the right is from 1785. Eilif Philipsen is dead, 103 years old "less 1 month and 1 day". City Archives of Bergen.

1640s it was much more difficult to get away with age exaggeration. People adjusted their behaviour accordingly, because few wanted to make fools of themselves. Apart from incurable mythomaniacs, only people coming from abroad or from other parts of the monarchy, first of all Norway and Schleswig, were seriously tempted to issue unsustained claims about their age.

How many, if any, of the nearly forty claims to an age of 100 years or more brought to the attention of Luxdorph by the Danish and Norwegian clergy can be sustained? Obviously all claims that cannot be sustained by some hard facts must be discarded. An absolute minimum requirement is a corresponding, well identified entry in a church register both for birth and death. Any further confirmation of their identity during their long lives is, of course, most welcome. Applying these basic criteria, all but one of the alleged centenarians in Luxdorph's material are invalidated. Most of them immediately, a couple after a few supplementary checks, including a woman called Margrethe Andersdatter, who was allegedly born in 1677 in Ingerslev Torup parish on the Island of Funen in a farming family and died at the age of 103 in Hjallese, Dalum parish, just outside Odense. A long biography of this fine woman is provided in a letter from a local clergyman, and everything sounds very reasonable and respectable, except perhaps for one detail: she claims that her mother obtained the very high age of 112. Anyway, Margrethe Andersdatter does not figure in the church register from 1677 of her alleged native parish. The information about the high age of her mother makes it tempting to suggest that perhaps she was one of those incurable mythomaniacs.

Eilif Philipsen - the first centenarian?

However, one is left, and that is the Norwegian, Eilif Philipsen from Ugenæs at Kinsarvik, near Bergen. He was christened together with his twin sister, Ingeborg, in Kinsarvik church on 21 July 1682. We know this for certain, because Kinsarvik was among the Norwegian parishes which on a voluntary basis kept a church register already in the 1670s. We come across him again in 1701, where he is mentioned in the first Norwegian census. He is here recorded as being 18 years old. At that time he lived with his father and two younger brothers, 10-year-old Jacob and 3-year-old Hans. Next time we see him is in 1721, where he is marrying the local 22-year-old Ingebjørk. We meet him again already two years later in 1723, when he was involved in a court case and in 1727, when he inherits his native farm. In 1753 at the age of 71 Eilif Philipsen handed over the farm to his son-in-law, the husband of his adopted daughter.

Then there is a gap of thirty years, before we meet him again. This time because he is mentioned in the local vicar's letter to Luxdorph. The vicar had taken a long time replying to Luxdorph's enquiry from 1780. He did not reply until April 1783. But then he also had something to tell, namely that there was a 101-year-old man in his parish. This was Eilif Philipsen, who still lived in retirement on his native farm together with his now 84-year-old wife. He lasted another two years. According to the church register in Kinsarvik Eilif Philipsen died 20 June 1785. There seems to be no doubt at all that the Eilif Philipsen, who died in Kinsarvik in 1785, was the very same Eilif Philipsen, who was christened at the same place almost 103 years earlier (Fig.5 and Fig. 6).

There is no doubt that Luxdorph cherished his collection of pictures much more than his statistical investigation from 1780. When he had visitors he loved to show them his collection of portraits of the old. It could be that as a contribution to the cultural history of old age and to the history of gerontology, the picture collection is of greater interest than the sociological material, contained in the replies from the Danish and Norwegian clergy to Luxdorph's letter of 1780 .

However, when we talk about centenarians, it is the 1780 investigation which counts. The picture gallery offers no serious candidate to an 18th century centenarian. The 1780 investigation does. Eilif Philipsen, by the way, seems to confirm the "tail theory", according to which centenarians do not emerge until well into the early-modern period. Not until the end of the 18th century, when the disease pattern in Europe had been less severe for quite a few decades, does it become time to look for the first centenarians. They may occur everywhere in Europe, so why not, indeed, in a well-to-do and socially stable rural district outside Bergen in Norway?

Literature

Kjærgaard, T. 1989. Bolle Willum Luxdorph's "longævi". About the earliest age research in Denmark. (In Danish). *Carlsbergfondets Årsskrift* 1989:124-35.

Kjærgaard, T. 1995. Eilif Philipsen - the first centenarian in Europe? (In Danish). *Gerontologi og Samfund* 11:1:4-5.

Danish Centenarians after 1800

by Axel Skytthe & Bernard Jeune

Many tales have been told about very old people, and the existence of centenarians has rarely been questioned. The number of reported centenarians through time, however, has been rather low until the middle of this century, when the number of centenarians increased dramatically (Kannisto 1994, Vaupel and Jeune, this monograph). Even though the number of reported centenarians in the past has been low, the reported ages at death of the oldest centenarians have been extremely high, e.g. the famous Danish-Norwegian sailor, Christian Drakenberg, who died in 1772 at the age of 146 (Bowerman 1939). The high ages of these very old centenarians have however been questioned by Thoms and others (Thoms 1873, Bowerman 1939, Ørberg 1972).

The highest probable age at the present level of mortality and the current size of the world's population is about 120 years for a woman (Kannisto and Thatcher 1993). This corresponds to the age of the oldest authenticated person in the world, Madame Jeanne Calment, who celebrated her 120th birthday in February 1995 (Allard et al. 1994). But if the mortality level is higher, and the population is smaller, as in older days, then the question arises: When did the first centenarian emerge? In this chapter we try to answer this question with regard to the emergence of the first Danish centenarian.

Data

Statistics on demographic data in Denmark are based on clerical registration in parish registers.

The first parish register appears at the beginning of the 17th century. In 1646 the King issued a decree by which the vicar in every parish was ordered to keep records of the date and the number of births, marriages and deaths in his parish. There were, however, no instructions on how the records were to be kept, and the quality of the records for the next 175 years varies. In 1812 a new decree stated that the registers should be kept in special pre-printed books with 7 different forms, including one for dead males and one for dead females. Since that year this has with a few minor changes been the standard for keeping records on births, marriages and deaths, although it took some years to introduce the forms all over the country (Ørberg 1982).

The collection of demographic data goes back to the 17th century. The collection was, however, sporadic and only carried out in some parts of Denmark. From 1735 reports on births and deaths from the parishes each year were sent to the central administration ("Commerce-kollegiet"). Until 1774 only the total number of deaths were reported, not in age categories. From 1775 to 1834 the number of deaths was given in 10 year age groups with "100 years and above" as the highest category, but the quality of the reported data was not very good. The instructions on how to count the deaths were not clear: Did 'the year' mean the calendar year or the ecclesiastical year. Furthermore, where should a person dying at the age of 80 be included - the category headings were "From 70 to 80 years" and "From 80 to 90 years".

Graduately the accuracy was improved by more detailed instructions on how to count the deaths. In 1835 the deaths were given in 5 year age groups, and from 1870 deaths were reported by single year of age with the exception that deaths at an age of 100 years or above still were reported as a total.

Since 1943 all deaths in Denmark are registered at DIKE (Danish Institute of Clinical Epidemiology) in a computerized form, and deaths can therefore be given by exact age after this year.

The first census in Denmark to report centenarians was in 1801, when 5 female centenarians were found. Censuses on a regular basis were held from 1834 with the next in 1840, and from that year a census was held every 5 or 10 years.

Before 1870 the census lists were completed by local civil servants in Copenhagen and other towns and by the vicar in the country. Only the head of a family had to go to the vicar and inform him about his family. From 1870 to 1930 each household or family in Copenhagen and towns had to complete a list of all persons in that family or household, while in the country the local parish council was in charge of completing the lists. From 1935 to 1970 the census lists were checked by the municipal public registers, which held information about every person living in a district (Det statistiske Departement 1966). In 1968 the CPR (Central Person Registry) person number system was introduced in Denmark, and the last paper-based census was held in 1970 (Danmarks Statistik 1994).

The collection and treatment of statistical and demographic data were in the hands of very few persons in the central administration until the middle of the 19th century. A separate office ("Tabelkontoret") was established i 1797, but it was closed in 1819 because of difficulties in making the required tables, internal arguments among staff members and the Danish national bankruptcy in 1814.

From 1834 to 1849 the collection and treatment of statistical data were administered by a commission with members from various offices of the central administration. The staff involved was rather small: In 1848 the staff included the 5 members of the commission and 6 scribes. The commission had to deal with all statistical requests, and demographic studies were only a part of their work. During the 1840's criticism from scientific statisticians increased, and this lead to the establishment of an independent office for treatment of statistical data in 1849 (Holck 1901).

The data used in this chapter on number of deaths and population were taken from published tables by Johansen (1975) (for the period 1775 - 1800), and from different published tables by the Statistical Office (Tabelkommisionen, Statistisk Bureau and Danmarks Statistik). Census counts were also taken from published tables by the Statistical Office. A complete list of the publications used can be obtained from the authors.

The estimates of population of centenarians on January 1st are taken from a database at Odense University on Danish mortality 1870-1992 (Skytthe et al. 1994). In this database populations over 80 are calculated by the extinct cohort method devised by Vincent (1951). From 1943 the number of deaths above 100 are given in exact ages, but before that year the age at death above 100 is estimated using the mortality rates of Sweden for the corresponding period.

Trends in the number of centenarians in Denmark 1775 - 1993

Table 1 shows the number of reported deaths of centenarians in Denmark since 1775 in groups of 10 years. In this 200-year period the Danish population increased from approximately 1 million to 5 million (Danmarks Statistik 1994). The numbers before 1801 are, however, minimum numbers, because data are missing for some parts of Denmark for certain years. It may therefore be assumed that the number of reported deaths of centenarians was over 100 per decade or in average over 10 per year in the period 1775-1814.

It is evident that the number of reported deaths of centenarians declines dramatically in first half of the 1800s from over 100 per decade to a minimum of 20-30 deaths per decade in the period 1854-94. This decline is especially evident for males. There are more reported female than male centenarians in all decades with a variation of the sex ratio between 1.4 and 5.6. The sex ratio is especially high in the period with the minimum of reported deaths among centenarians.

Table 1: Danish Centenarians since 1775

Period	Females	Males	Total	Sex ratio F : M
1775-1784	49	28	77	1.75
1785-1794	62	34	96	1.82
1795-1804	77	20	97	3.85
1805-1814	74	51	125	1.45
1815-1824	52	34	86	1.53
1825-1834	64	28	92	2.29
1835-1844	24	16	40	1.50
1845-1854	31	17	48	1.82
1855-1864	22	9	31	2.44
1865-1874	16	3	19	5.33
1875-1884	22	6	28	3.67
1885-1894	22	6	28	3.67
1895-1904	34	9	43	3.78
1905-1914	39	7	46	5.57
1915-1924	31	12	43	2.58
1925-1934	48	23	71	2.09
1935-1944	53	32	85	1.66
1945-1954	85	48	133	1.77
1955-1964	119	87	206	1.37
1965-1974	218	103	321	2.12
1975-1984	600	257	857	2.33
1985-1992	955	324	1279	2.95
Total	2697	1154	3851	2.34

This decline in the first half of the 1800s is also evident when the number of reported deaths of centenarians is calculated per million population - from over 10 to under 2 per million (see Figure 1). Figure 1 also shows population data on centenarians since 1870 when we had the possibility of estimating the number of

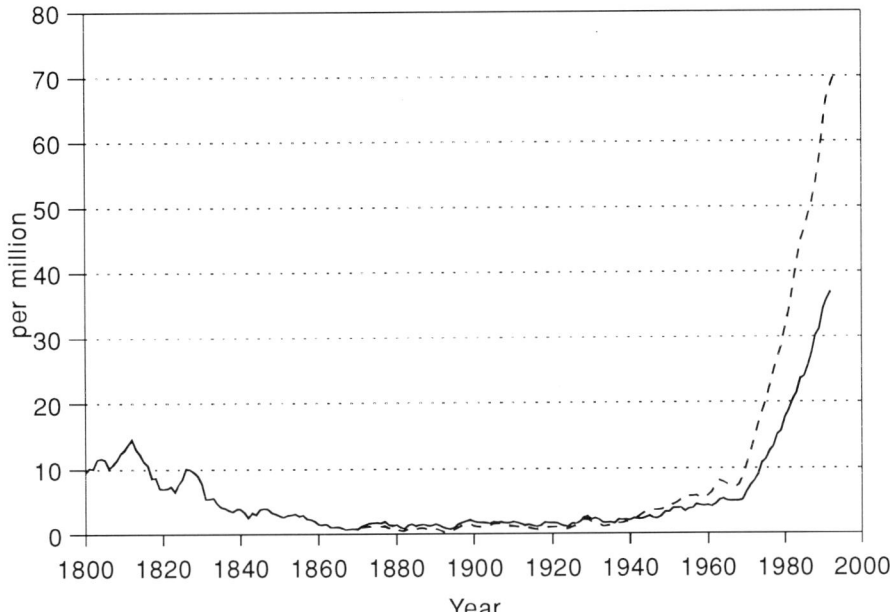

Figure 1: Centenarians per million population in Denmark 1800-1993. Full line: reported deaths. Dotted line: estimated number of centenarians Jan 1. Five years moving average.

living centenarians per year based on Vincent's extinct cohort method (Vincent 1951). It shows that the number of estimated living centenarians did not exceed the number of reported deaths of centenarians until 1940.

The level of centenarians seems almost constant in the period from 1860 to 1930. From around 1965 the number of centenarians increases tremendously to a number of 73 per million in 1993. In this last period the estimated number of living centenarians increases faster than the number of deaths of centenarians, ending with a twofold difference. This rapid development reflects the decrease of the mortality rate of centenarians shown by Kannisto (1994).

Figure 2 shows three different ways of illustrating the number of centenarians in the period 1800 to 1960. The filled squares represent census reporting of the number of centenarians per million. The number of centenarians reported at censuses shows a dramatic fall in a very narrow period from 1845 to 1860 and continued decline to 1900.

It is hard to believe that this decline is due to deterioration of living conditions; industrialisation in Denmark only began slowly in the latter half of the 1800s. A plausible explanation is a more careful validation of the reported ages at census after the establishment of Statistisk Bureau in 1849. Understanding the importance of

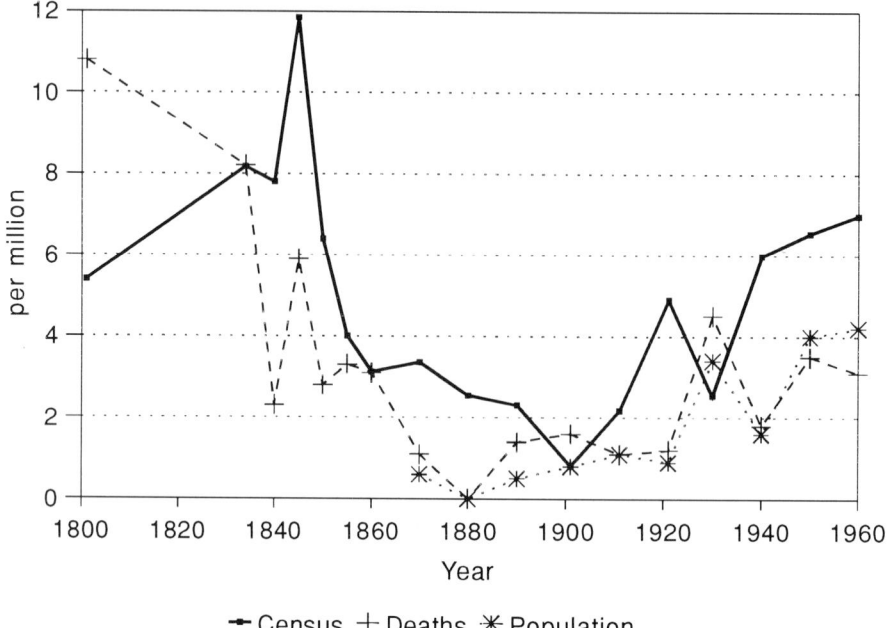

Figure 2 Three different estimates of Danish centenarians per million population 1800-1960. Census count (■). Reported number of deaths (+). Estimated centenarian population (✳).

correct data and awareness may also have contributed to a more careful registration of age, when the census lists were filled, and also when a death was reported to the local vicar.

The third curve, represented by stars, shows estimates of the centenarian population on January 1 based on the extinct cohort method. The difference between the estimated population and the census count could in part be due to the fact that the mortality rates used in calculation of deaths when these were not reported were taken from Swedish data. But it could also be a consequence of over-reporting of centenarians in the censuses due to age-exaggeration.

Though we only have estimates of the population of centenarians on 1 January, the following 2 figures are based on these, because this is the best available measure of the prevalence of centenarians at a given time.

On the basis of the estimated number of centenarians from different periods three exponential regression lines were fitted (Figure 3). Assuming an increase in the population size which in itself could explain an increase in centenarians, each regression line has been extrapolated backward in time to where it crosses 1 centenarian. This would give an indication of the year when the first centenarian emerged in Denmark if the conditions had been the same earlier as in the period the

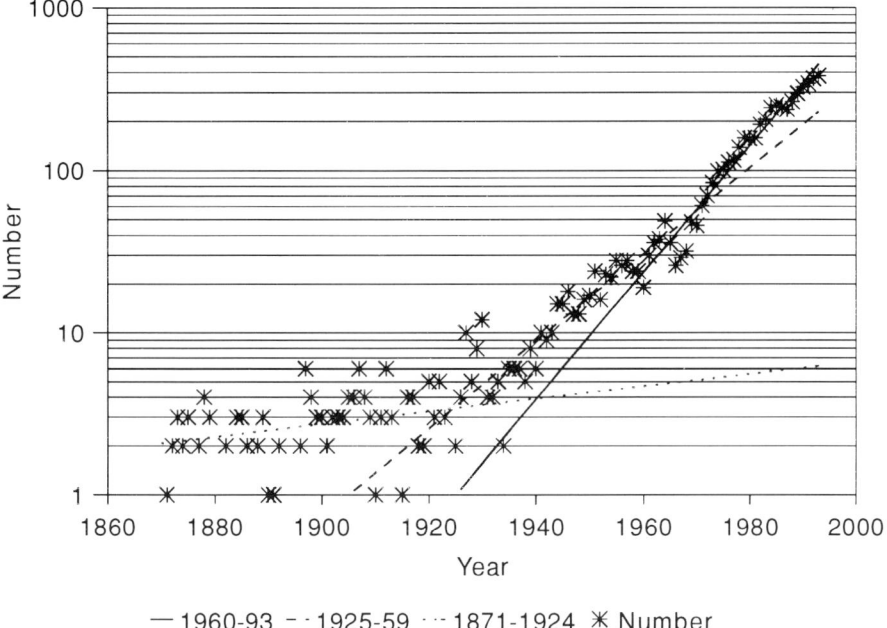

Figure 3 Calculated number of centenarians on 1 Jan. 1870-1992. The 3 regression lines are based on different periods. Note the logarithmic scale on the Y-axis.

regression is based on.

If the fit is based on the period from 1925-59, the first centenarian would have emerged after 1900 (i.e. 1905). Accepting the population estimates as being correct and assuming that the increase from 1870 to 1924, which as shown earlier is very slow, corresponds with the "natural" increase in the last century, then extrapolation back in time would indicate the "true" year of the first centenarian. This year turns out to be year 1795, in good correspondence with the deliberately provocative allegation - no centenarians before year 1800, at least in Denmark - which was proposed before this analysis was done (Jeune 1994).

Assuming that the extrapolated curve in Figure 4 represents the true trend in centenarians, most of the reported deaths as centenarians in the hundred year period 1760-1860 must have been assigned too high an age at death.

The Danish Centenarian Registry

We have decided to establish a database of Danish centenarians with a verified age in order to determine the exact proliferation of centenarians in modern time and to

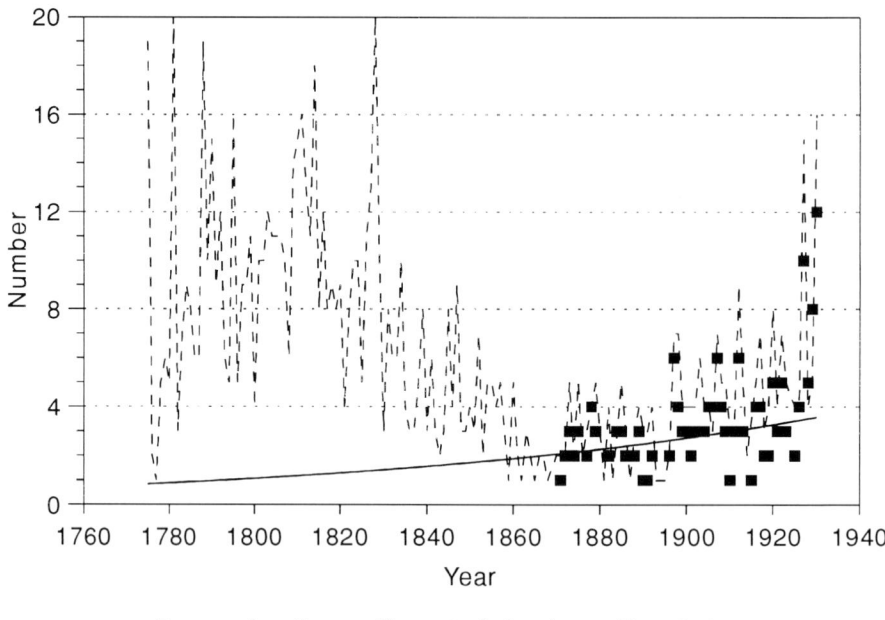

Figure 4: Number of reported dead centenarians 1775-1930 with the extrapolated regression line based on the estimates of centenarian population 1871-1924.

determine when the first 100-year-old individual, the first 101-year-old, the first 102-year-old, etc. emerged in Denmark. At this moment we only know that the first verified 110-year-old woman emerged in Denmark on 26 November 1994.

The identification of centenarians is central in establishing the database. As a starting point we use the number, given in the published statistics of deaths, with an age of 100 years or higher as a key to how many centenarians we expect to find each year. Each alleged centenarian has then to be identified. This is an easy task as far as the last 50 years are concerned. From the Central Person Registry it is possible to identify all living centenarians, and also those who have died since 1 April 1968. Further, the Death Certificate Registry at DIKE, which was started in 1943, includes all dead centenarians since 1943.

But prior to that time it is more difficult. No easy way to identify centenarians before 1943 exists. From the beginning of the 19th century to 1868 and a single year 1887, the original reports of number of births, marriages and deaths which were sent from the parishes to the Statistical Bureau exist in the National Archives ("Rigsarkivet") in Copenhagen. By carefully going through these it is possible to locate the parishes that reported dead centenarians, and then check the death (or burial) registers from these parishes.

Table 2 : Sources for identification of centenarians

Sources for identification of centenarians	
From 1968	Central person register (CPR)
From 1943	Death certificate register (DIKE)
Approx. 1800 - 1868 and 1887	Original reports from parishes to the Statistical Bureau
From approx. 1650 - 1890	Indexes on deaths at some regional archives
1890 - 1942	Difficult ! No yearly reports available, only census lists

In each of the 4 regional archives, where the parish registers are archived, indexes on marriages and deaths exist for some of the parishes, covering the period from beginning of the parish register, about 1650-1700, to about 1890. By looking through these indexes it is possible to catch almost every alleged centenarian up to 1891. This has been done for approximately 3/4 of the parishes in the county of Funen, where indexes exist. Parish registers for the remaining 1/4 of parishes were searched, resulting in a total of 275 reported centenarians. Assuming that Funen corresponds to 1/8 of the Danish population at any time, this would indicate a total number of 2,200 alleged centenarians before 1890 in Denmark.

For the years between 1891 and 1942 it is necessary to rely on the kind cooperation of other people. We have contacted genealogists, local historical archives in Denmark and others, who might know anything about very old people.

Until now we have focused on the period 1848 - 68, mainly because of the existence of the original reports, but also because this is the period where the number of reported centenarians is about the same as indicated by the extrapolated curve.

Approximately 5,000 alleged centenarians are expected to be included in the database. Of these 2,400 have been recorded as centenarians since 1968, and approximately 500 are from the period 1835 - 1942. Until now (Dec. 1994) we have identified approximately 350 alleged centenarians before 1943, so we still have some work to do.

Table 3 : Four levels of certainty of age

Verification of Age	
Level	Criteria
D	Death date and age (no verification)
C	Birth registration
B	Life story
A	Family reconstructed

A very important aspect of establishing the database is to verify the age of alleged centenarians. As an indicator of how well documented the age is, we use 4 levels of certainty of the age. The lowest level, D, is simply a reported age of 100 years or more. This is, of course, insufficient. As a minimum the birth (or baptism) must be documented by a registration in a parish register; this is level C.

It is, however, still necessary to have more information in order to verify the age with certainty. You must be able to reconstruct at least part of the life history of the person with data from other sources such as appearance in census lists, confirmation, military service etc. A verification at this level is classified as level B.

In order to be sure of avoiding any namesakes, it is in addition necessary to find all brothers and sisters because of a fairly common practice of naming a newborn baby after a predeceased brother or sister. Thoms gave several examples of this in his book (Thoms 1873), and Johansen (1975) has also observed this in his work on the Danish population in the 18th and 19th century.

If we want to follow Thoms "species of evidence" we must therefore go to the highest level of verification, level A, which requires the total reconstruction of the family of the centenarian, i.e. date of birth and death of both parents, their wedding date, the name and date of birth and deaths of all brothers and sisters. All these data must be found and checked which is very time-consuming.

The verification of age is a slow process compared to the identification. However, at the identification we attempt to verify the age to at least level C. Verification to level B is often possible because of the possibility of using census lists in order to find the place of birth.

The intention is to verify all centenarians, who died in the period 1835 to 1943, to at least level B. If verification to this level is satisfactory, we will consider the person in question as a true centenarian, knowing the possibility that we might include some false centenarians due to namesaking. Centenarians, who died after 1943, will in general be considered as true centenarians, when they are verified to level C. We consider the information in the Death Register at DIKE as being valid because of the long-standing tradition for registration of demographic events in Denmark. However if we find any difference in the number of centenarians reported by the official statistics and the number reported from DIKE, every individual dying that year will be checked and verified to at least level B.

Verifying the age of an alleged centenarian before 1840 is increasingly difficult, partly because of the quality of information in parish registers, partly because of an increasing probability that parish registers do not exist, when you go back to the eighteenth and seventeenth century, mainly lost due to fires at the vicar's residence. Finally it can be very difficult to locate the place of birth, when there is no supplementary information from, for instance, censuses.

The top level verification is very expensive to do and will not be done on all alleged centenarians, but only on those at extreme ages (the 5 or 10 oldest centenarians each year as well as all above 105 in the whole period and centenarians above 103 before 1940).

Finally an example of the verification process: In a little parish on Fyn, Rorslev near Middelfart, a man by the name Mads Pedersen Ribe died 24 April 1864 at the age of 109 years. Obviously the vicar also thought that this was an extreme age, because in the burial register he added "Born in Ribe 24 June 1755". Looking in the parish register for Ribe Cathedral we do find an entry saying " .. 24 June 1755 Mads, son of Peder Madsen, soldier". But that is all. There is simply no information on his mother.

Furthermore - it is not possible to find Mads Pedersen Ribe in any of the census lists from the parish in the period 1834-60. This means that either he has arrived at the parish after 1860 - at the alleged age of 105 - or he has lived as a recluse without contact to others for many years. In the probate register it is stated "Pauper Mads Pedersen Ribe has died at the age of 109 - no possessions, no information about heirs". Thus the status of Mads Pedersen Ribe as a centenarian can only be verified to level C. This is not sufficient to consider Mads Pedersen Ribe a true centenarian.

Literature

Allard, M., V. Lèbre, and J.M. Robine. 1994. Les 120 ans de Jeanne Calment. Documents. *Le Cherche Midi Editeur*, Paris.

Bowerman, W.G. 1939. Centenarians. *Transactions of the Actuarial Society of America* 40:360-378.

Danmarks Statistik. 1905. Population conditions in Denmark in the 19th century. (in Danish). *Statistisk Tabelværk VA*, 5. København,

Danmarks Statistik. 1994a. Statistical Yearbook 1994. København.

Danmarks Statistik. 1994b. Vital Statistics 1992. København.

Holck, A. 1901. History of Danish Statistics 1800-1850. (in Danish) *Statens Statistiske Bureau*, København.

Jeune, B. 1994. Centenarians - tail or tale? (in Danish). *Gerontologi og Samfund* 10: 4-6.

Johansen, H.C. 1975. Population development and family structure in the 18th century. (in Danish) *Odense University Press*, Odense.

Kannisto, V. 1994. Development of Oldest-Old Mortality. 1950-1990: Evidence from 28 Developed Countries. *Odense University Press*, Odense.

Kannisto, V., and A.R. Thatcher. 1993. The plausibility of certain reported cases of extreme longevity. *Manuscript*.

Skytthe, A., K. Andreev, and U. Larsen. 1994. The Danish mortality database at Odense University 1870-1992. Documentation. *Manuscript*.

Det Statistiske Departement. 1966. Population studies and health conditions 1901-1960. (in Danish) *Statistiske undersøgelser nr 19*. København.

Thoms, W.J. 1873. Human Longevity. Its Facts and Its Fictions. *John Murray*, London.

Vincent, P. 1951. La mortalité des vieillards. *Population* 6:181-204.

Ørberg, P. 1972. Petite Drakenberg studies. (in Danish) *Personalhistorisk Tidsskrift* 1972:270-273.

Ørberg, P. 1982. Churchbooks and churchbook politics 1812-1920. (in Danish) *Samlinger 1982*, p.125-164.

Record Longevity in Swedish Cohorts Born since 1700

by Hans Lundström

People reaching an unusually high age have always been of particular interest. This is especially true for those who attained the age of 100 or more. Many tales have been told about very old people in Sweden. We can take Jon Andersson as an example. He died 18 April 1729. According to the death register he was born 18 February 1582. This means he was no less than 147 years old at death. This high age was of course commented upon and Jon was said to be the oldest person in Sweden ever where the age could be verified (Valentin 1966). Another example is Nils Öhrberg who died 12 October 1816, 116 years old according to the death register. He was married three times. Nils seems to have survived both wives and children. He was a sexton until the age of 108 when he had to retire (Valentin 1966). There are many more tales like these about persons who got very old.

The question is to what extent data on age can be relied upon. A person living to the age of 147 is of course impossible, especially as far back in time as 1729. The oldest authenticated person ever in the world is Madame Jeanne Calment. She passed her 120th birthday in February 1995. A person 116 years old at the beginning of the 19th century seems impossible too. There are many more persons reported as more than 100 years old at death during the 1749-1900 period. In this chapter I will try to answer the question how reliable the Swedish population data really are.

The church registers as base for population statistics

For more than 300 years each parish in Sweden has kept a complete and continually updated register of its population. From 1686 it was compulsory for each parish to keep registers on births, deaths, migration, marriages and divorces as well as a population register. In some parishes this registration had started long before 1686. In other parishes the registration seems to have started at a later date.

Apart from the usual church registers Sweden had a very special register, "husförhörslängden" (the catechetical examination register). This register was originally introduced to keep track of literacy, understanding of the bible and other facts of interest to the clergy. This register after some time turned into a full-fledged population register including all persons living in the parish. Just like a census the register was arranged by household. Among other facts the date of birth was registered for each person. What makes the register very special is the fact that it was continuously updated. That is, the general population registered showed the actual population (de jure) living in the parish at any time (providing that the clergy updated the register regularly as they were supposed to do).

The various church registers were tightly linked. When a birth was registered the child was entered in the population register too. When a person moved out of the parish the migration was registered in the migration register, and he was removed from the population register. From time to time the clergy made some mistakes. Some, if not most, of these errors were detected in the yearly updates of the taxation register. Quality in the church registers gradually improved and by 1860 data can be considered as virtually correct. One reason for this was the rising interest in population matters among scholars and the general public. The clergy became aware of the importance of keeping the registers accurately. Another reason was the very strict control of all statistics that was introduced in 1860. The compilation of population statistics was from that year and onwards carried out by Statistics Sweden. The compilation was based on copies of all parish registers sent to Statistics Sweden. This made it possible for the first time to make a very careful check of all data. When in doubt the local parish was contacted and data corrected if necessary. Age was for the first time centrally calculated based on register information. The only remaining problem was, and still is, that all migration was not registered. In principle we have the same kind of base for the population statistics today as we had in 1749. In 1946 population registration was made a concern of the state. The church continued to keep the base, the local registers of the population up to 1991 when this task was taken over by the local tax offices. The system was computerised in 1967 and the introduction of personal identity numbers in 1947 made the computerisation efficient.

Quality of age data

The special interest in the oldest old can be seen in the statistical tables. When the collection of population statistics started in 1749, deaths were to be reported in five-year age groups up to the age of 90. For all 90 years of age or older each death had to be specified by age and sex in a special part of the form reserved for comments. It was not uncommon that the clergy added to these more detailed facts a short memoir of the deceased. That is, detailed information on centenarians is available in Sweden for a period of more than 240 years.

For the 1749-1859 period population statistics were put together in each parish. The clergy was responsible for this task and they used information from the church registers. Before the statistical tables were sent to the forerunner of Statistics Sweden they passed several authorities. The parish tables were sent to the rectorial district where data for all parishes were summarised into one table for the rectorial district. That table in turn was sent to the rural deanery and so on. In this process some information naturally can have been left out. Especially extra comments that were not explicitly asked for can have disappeared in this process. According to Lublin (1957), however, the county tables seem to include most if not all comments and detailed information of those who were 90 years of age or older. However, it was not quite clear how to fill in the form. Deaths were to be reported in five-year age classes. The classes were of the form ...75-79,80-85, 85-90. Was a person who was exactly 90 years old at death to be reported in the 85-90 age group or not? This possible source of misunderstanding was more or less eliminated in 1774 when new forms were introduced. From 1802 there was no longer room for any misunderstandings. The five-year age groups 0-5,5-10 .. up to 95-100 asked for, were in the table followed by the one-year age groups 101,102 ... up to 115. A person exactly 100 years old was no longer by mistake added to the 95-100 age group but to the 101 group (100 up to but not including age 101).

Apart from misunderstandings over how to use the table resulting in minor errors the more serious error remained. At least up to 1786 the clergy had rarely, if ever, information in the registers on date of birth for centenarians who died. The deceased were born before 1686 when registration of all births in a special birth register started. In order to calculate age the clergy had to rely on information from relatives only. This of course meant that the reported age at death was sometimes exaggerated, especially for very old persons. The table below shows both the absolute number of centenarians and the relative number per 1 million of the total population for the 1751-1990 period.

According to the official statistics the number of deceased centenarians was very high in the 1750s. The absolute number of deaths as well as the relative number then decreased to a minimum around 1835 and then slowly started to increase again. This development is not what one would expect and clearly indicates an error in data.

Table 1: Centenarians deceased 1751-1990

Period	Number	Per 1 million of total population
1751-1760	449	24
1761-1770	252	13
1771-1780	160	8
1781-1790	155	7
1791-1800	82	4
1801-1810	75	4
1811-1820	38	2
1821-1830	56	2
1831-1840	31	1
1841-1850	32	1
1851-1860	30	1
1861-1870	34	1
1871-1880	43	1
1881-1890	43	1
1891-1900	63	1
1901-1910	75	2
1911-1920	154	3
1921-1930	252	4
1931-1940	303	5
1941-1950	275	4
1951-1960	374	5
1961-1970	584	8
1971-1980	1156	14
1981-1990	2412	29

Source: Lublin 1957 and Befolkningsförändringar 1956-1990

According to the table there were twice as many deceased centenarians in the first 50-year period as in the following 100-year period. Furthermore, in the 1751-1800 period 99 of the deceased were registered as 108 years old or older. The maximum age at death was as high as 127 (Lublin 1957). Assuming the same relative number of deceased centenarians as in the mid 1850s there would have been only some 100 deaths at the most in the 1751-99 period instead of 1098.

Census data show a similar pattern with a high proportion of persons aged 90 or more in 1750 declining up to 1800 (Figure 1). This fact with a high proportion

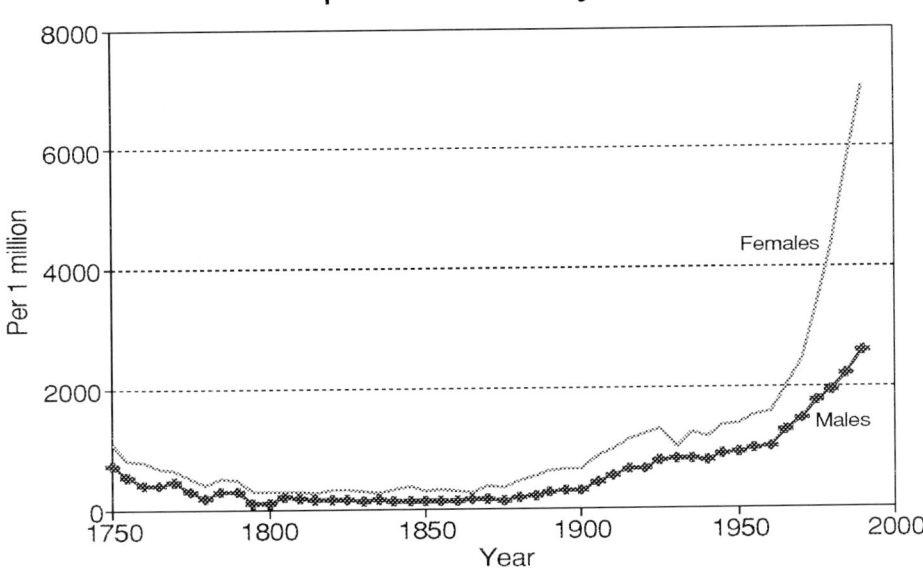

Figure 1
Source: Sundbärg 1903, BiSOS various years, Befolkningsförändringar 1911-90.

of old people in the middle of the 18th century was commented upon in a statistical report some 100 years later. It was said that there could have been some mistakes when registering the age as many persons were born before the keeping of church registers had started. Comparing with other countries, however, Statistics Sweden found that Norway had very high rates. This was taken as an indication that the Swedish data might not be so wrong after all (BiSOS 1851-55 Del 3 p.25). This is of course not true. There are clear errors in the data. This was also pointed out by Sundbärg (1903).

Using the extinct cohort method for the 1820-60 period the official population size can be compared with the calculated population aged 90+. The calculations clearly show that there was some kind of error in the data (Table 2). The difference between official and calculated population size indicates errors in the official population size and in age at death. Persons who had disappeared from the parish some time ago or perhaps had died were still included in the population register. The explanation for this error is the tightly linked registers. As no death or migration was reported the population register was not updated. This error was not taken care of until 1870 with the introduction of a register of 'residence unknown'. When the whereabouts of a person was unknown he was after some time entered in the register of 'residence unknown' and his name was taken off the population register.

Table 2: **Official and calculated number of persons 90+ using the extinct cohort method**

	Males		Females	
	Official	Calculated	Official	Calculated
1820	191	201	424	449
1830	193	165	435	371
1840	193	197	536	427
1850	211	177	532	435

Calculation based number of deaths by age in five-year age groups.

Verifying age at death

In the individual cases the only way to check the age is to find register information of some kind, for example registration in the birth register. For the period 1860 to 1992 it is not necessary to verify age at death as that has already been done by Statistics Sweden. From 1907 a list of all centenarians was published yearly with information on name, date of birth, age at death and other facts for each individual. For census years a list of all centenarians was published too with detailed information about each person. It is only the death of Dorothea Andersdotter in 1860 that may be questioned. She was registered as 110 years old at death but in the copy of the church register age was just given in years and not as in all other cases specified in months and days too.

For the period before 1860 there are certainly a number of deaths where the stated age is not correct (Figure 2). The quality of data seems to deteriorate as we go back in time. There is a clear change in pattern of deaths by age before and after 1860. In the 1816-59 period there are many observations of very old persons, a pattern that changed abruptly in 1860. Furthermore there was a concentration of persons 100 years of age at death in the 1816-35 period clearly indicating some error in data. The only way to check age at death is to track down each individual, trying to find the person in the church registers. This is a very time-consuming method. You probably end up with certain authenticated centenarians and others who probably

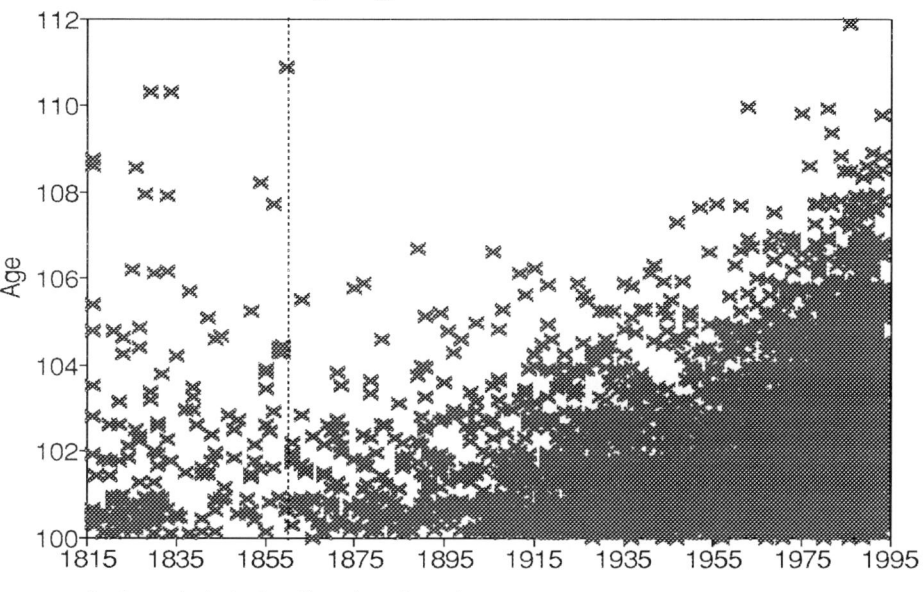

Figure 2

were as old as the clergy registered in the death register. For all other deaths nothing can be said at all. For those who died before 1800 and were said to be 100 years old or older it is highly unlikely that age can be verified at all.

The only thing that could be completed was a list of all deaths 1816-59 with information on year of death, age at death, sex and in which parish the death occurred - information which has not been readily available before. This list can form the starting point for a more thorough search of the parish registers.

The question when the first centenarian emerged in Sweden cannot be answered as yet. Only very uncertain speculations are possible at this time indicating that the first centenarian in Sweden perhaps emerged in the 1820s or 1830s.

The age record in Sweden

The oldest old female in Sweden ever registered and verified was a woman called Hulda who died in 1994, 112 years and 105 days old. The second oldest woman died in 1986 and was 111 years 2 months and 28 days old. The oldest male in Sweden ever registered and verified was Nikolaus who died in 1993, 109 years and 236 days old.

Literature

Arosenius, E. 1928. Bidrag till det svenska tabellverkets historia. Stockholm.

Befolkningsförändringar. *Yearly publication on vital statistics 1911-92.*

BiSOS A. Bidrag till Sveriges Officiella Statistik. A. Befolkningsstatistik. *Statistiska centralbyrån.* Stockholm. /Annual reports 1851 to 1910./

Hofsten, E., and H. Lundström. 1976. Swedish Population history. Main trends from 1750 to 1970. In Urval. *No 8 Statistiska centralbyrån.* Stockholm.

Kangas, U. 1986. Mortalitets- och folkmängdstabeller. Källbeskrivning. *Demografiska databasen.* Umeå.

Lublin, F. 1957. Svenska hundraåringar under två århundranden. In *Statistisk tidskrift No 5.* Stockholm.

Nilsdotter, J.U. 1993. Parish records. 19th Century Ecclesiastical Registers. In *Information from the Demographic Data Base.* Umeå.

Sundbärg, G. 1903. Rikets folkmängd åren 1750-1900, fördelad efter ålder och kön. In *Statistisk Tidskrift 1903 No 2.*

Sundbärg, G. 1905. Döde efter kön, ålder och civilstånd i Sverige åren 1751-1900 samt medelfolkmängden efter kön och ålder under femårsperioderna för samma tid. In *Statistisk Tidskrift 1905 No 2.*

Sundbärg, G. 1907. Bevölkerungsstatistik Schwedens 1750-1900. Einige Hauptresultate. Stockholm :1907. Reprint: *Urval No 3* . Stockholm 1970/.

Tabellkommissionens underdåniga berättelser. Various years 1816 - 1856.

Tabellverket. Annual statistical reports on microfiche 1749-1859. Riksarkivet.

Valentin, A. 1966. Sveriges 100-åringar. Stockholm.

Personal communications with representatives from local archives and the Demographic Database in Umeå.

The Oldest Old in Pre-Industrial Britain: Centenarians before 1800 - Fact or Fiction?

by Julia Hynes

Vaupel and Jeune (in this monograph) argue that because of the high death rates prevalent in the past, most accounts of centenarians in earlier centuries must be inaccurate. Like many others, these authors are sceptical about the reliability of reported longlivers, particularly those supposedly dying aged at least one hundred before the start of the 19th century. Kannisto (1988) vented similar concerns when he wrote, *"The major problem of statistics relating to centenarians is that they are vulnerable to age errors. There is a general tendency to overstate the ages of old persons as they and their family members take pride in their alleged longevity. This tendency is more pronounced in populations that are not accustomed to keeping records of age and often results in fanciful claims to extreme longevity in countries in which there was no birth registration at the time when the persons in question were born"*.

The aim of this study is to prove beyond reasonable doubt that individuals did live into their eleventh decade in England and Wales in the era before the demographic transition, that is, before the 19th century. If this aim can be fulfilled, this study will have substantial implications for current research that is focusing on present and future, rather than historical maximal length of life.

For example, assumptions about the aging process among humans might be revised because the evidence will indicate that in a high mortality regime and adverse environment, some individuals, albeit in small numbers, can survive to ages which even today, are considered to be very old. In their article "Reductions in Mortality at Advanced Ages", Kannisto et al. (1993) wrote, *"The traditional view is that a single, universal process of aging produces an exponential increase in mortality with age - the law Gompertz published in 1825 - and that "like a clock" every individual "is constructed to run a certain time". The current evidence, together with the results presented here, suggests a new paradigm of aging that recognizes a rich variety of diverse and often highly plastic aging processes that can be influenced by health interventions, behavioural changes, and environmental improvements and that depend on genetic differences both between and within species"*. The results of this study might support this new paradigm of aging.

Unfortunately, results of statistical modelling used to estimate the probability of individuals living to become centenarians in the high mortality regime of the past show that the chances of survival into the eleventh decade of life were extremely small before 1800. Consequently, those few people who did survive substantially beyond the mean age at death are usually believed to be untrue because statistically they are highly improbable. However, if some reports of extreme longevity can be confirmed, those sceptical of the existence of the unusually long lived before the start of the 19th century may have to modify their views.

Secondly, if centenarians are verified in a high mortality regime, there are substantial implications for potential maximal length of life span in the present and future low mortality regime, which has a healthier environment and which is supported by highly developed medical treatment. The observed increase in maximal length of life between 1800 and 1994 might be deemed less than presently thought and certainly less than the overall mortality decline.

Thirdly, if the maximum verified age at death has not risen by the same degree to which general adult mortality has declined, the study might provide support for the argument that there is indeed a biological maximal length of life and although it has not yet been reached, it is being approached by an increasing number of people in today's lower mortality regime.

In order for these implications to be developed further, it must be shown that centenarians existed in the pre-industrial poor environmental, low technology, high mortality era. This is not an easy task because compulsory registration of vital events did not begin in England and Wales until 1537; consequently, mass observation of the population is not possible until the early 16th century. Using figures estimated by Wrigley and Schofield (1981), from 1537 to 1800 there were between 22 and 25 million people in England of whom only a small number, perhaps 900, could possibly have been centenarians at their death. Unfortunately, as it only became compulsory to record age at death in parish registers in 1812 many surviving burial registers lack age at death information, making it especially difficult to locate potential centenarians dying before 1800. Consequently, family reconstitution studies and published potted biographies must be the main source of age at death information when researching the mortality of large groups in the period before the introduction of civil registration in 1837. Although the number of people included in such studies are only a small proportion of the potential 22 to 25 million, so long as a single centenarian can be reasonably confirmed to have died before 1800, the aim of this study will have been fulfilled.

Verifying reported centenarians - some problems

It will be revealed below how difficult this task is for the period before civil registration began, mainly due to the lack of surviving records. Although there are numerous studies and publications providing details of long-livers in the past all the way back to the ancient Greeks and Romans, few reports are substantiated (Bailey 1857, Weber 1914, Ernest 1938, Parkin 1992). Indeed most rely on the notoriously inaccurate tombstone inscription or age at death information written in parish burial registers. Others readily accept recollections, usually false, of famous events as proof of the age of an elderly individual or a frequently inaccurate estimate of the age at death of the corpse. Hence, because systematic record keeping was both less frequent and less reliable before the introduction in 1837 of civil registration in England and Wales and because positively linking the birth/baptismal, marriage and death records, which may exist, to an individual requires additional evidence which is dependent on the "visibility" of the person in other surviving records; identifying a true centenarian is a complex process. However, this should not deter the researcher because, to quote Parkin (1992), *"Comparative evidence tells us that the number of alleged centenarians in Roman Africa is a gross exaggeration. But that is not to say that some people did not survive the century mark and beyond"*. Consequently, although many reported centenarians throughout history up to the present day are undoubtedly incorrect, some are true; these individuals must be identified and verified.

Unfortunately, when attempting to verify probable centenarians, those chosen are not randomly selected, mainly because those in the "Maximal Length of Life" project's database are biased towards the male elite in British society, but also because certain groups are likely to have more surviving records facilitating a life history to be constructed. Those at extreme ends of the spectrum, the wealthy, public figures or paupers are more likely to be featured in records other than vital events which help to build up a picture of the life course of the individual. In the case of the privileged, documentation survives especially for males because they were more likely to attend university, enter a profession or business, later feature in public life in an official capacity and ultimately make a will which was proved upon death. In contrast their wives were likely to remain in quiet obscurity, precluding them from records. However, diaries of middle and upper class ladies are a possible source of evidence to support a claim from one of their number of being a centenarian at death.

As both male and female paupers appeared in "poor law" records when receiving financial assistance, which lends support to reported death dates and age at death information for the poor in pre-nineteenth century Britain, in some instances less privileged members of society are as well documented, and so traceable, as their wealthier counterparts.

In contrast, an individual who was neither extremely rich nor extremely poor and was not renowned at a local or national level was probably less frequently recorded and consequently more difficult to trace throughout his/her career.

However, because verification of a reported centenarian is the primary goal of this chapter, selection and bias are peripheral problems which will only affect the type of person likely to be chosen for attempted verification.

Criteria for successful verification

Thoms (1873), an informed nineteenth century sceptic of reports of extremely long lived individuals, stated that when a centenarian is being verified, *"the proof of it should be clear, distinct, and beyond dispute"*. He has shown many reports of extreme longevity to be false and questioned the use of individual pieces of evidence from the most popular sources; baptismal certificates, tombstone inscriptions, the number of the Centenarian's descendants, the recollections of the Centenarian and the evidence of old people still living who knew the Centenarian as 'very old' when they themselves were quite young. Thoms (1879) believed additional corroborative evidence such as the dates of birth, surname and christian name of the individual's father and mother, the place and date of their marriage, the birth dates of any brothers or sisters, the date of the "potential" centenarian's marriage and of the births of his/her children, the dates of his/her admission to school, entrance into the army, navy or any other public employment or apprenticeship, all to be essential. Unfortunately, the above criteria could be viewed as too rigorous and unrealistic because as made clear above, only very rarely indeed could centenarians dying before 1800 who have all the evidence Thoms recommends be located, primarily due to the small number of extremely long-lived in observation and inadequate survival or initial compilation of relevant records. It must be borne in mind that many reported centenarians checked by Thoms were his contemporaries. Consequently, access to relevant information and documents was rather easier than attempting the same verification procedure one hundred years later when some records will have been lost or destroyed and relations or close descendants are no longer available to discuss the person in question.

However, failure to locate a relevant record should not necessarily disqualify the candidate from the list of potentially verifiable centenarians. A degree of flexibility and the use of judgement after the presentation of all the evidence is surely essential when seeking a centenarian dying before 1800. Hence, guidelines detailing the degree of probability of the individual being a true centenarian according to the records and combination of records acquired, rather than rules specifying certainty should be introduced because finding enough evidence to verify a centenarian beyond dispute has to be deemed an unrealistic task in most cases. For instance, if there is no birth/baptismal record for a potential centenarian but there is a flourishing date at which an age can be confidently estimated, the calculated birth date should be accepted. Alternatively, if a long-liver has an unusual name and has a birth/baptismal and a death/burial date but has large periods of time when no information is available concerning their activities, as long as potential confusion with name-sakes can be discounted, then the individual's reported vital event dates should be accepted despite lack of supporting evidence for significant periods of time. Perhaps a set of guidelines and probabilities of a person being a centenarian at death according to the available evidence and competing name-sakes should be established along similar lines to family reconstitution linkage introduced by Wrigley and Schofield. This would enable individuals with less than ideal evidence to be allotted a probability level of being a centenarian.

Reported and calculated centenarians in the maximal length of life database: Case studies of attempted verification

The "potential" centenarians dying before the start of the nineteenth century whose life histories will be checked for authenticity originate from the data accumulated in the "Maximal Length of Life" project (table 1). This information was collected to analyse the whole old age mortality curve during the centuries leading up to the demographic transition rather than for the specific purpose of the verification of "potential" centenarians. It follows that there are probably "potential" centenarians who are more easily verifiable but who do not appear in these particular datasets collected for the analysis of historical old age mortality.

    An important distinction has to be made between "reported" and "calculated" centenarians in the database. "Reported" centenarians are those old people whose age at death is stated to be at least one hundred. The report might be a written statement of age at death in the parish register, on an individual's tombstone or it might be a newspaper obituary notice. In many instances, these reported cases cannot be substantiated due to the absence of additional information. However, the evidence for "calculated" centenarians is more robust because they are identified from the summation of their age at death using their stated birth/baptism and death/burial dates. Hence, there are two pieces of information from which the search for additional evidence can begin.

The datasets forming the *"Maximal Length of Life"* database on age at death of individuals between the sixteenth and twentieth centuries can be divided into two, those with "reported" and those with "calculated" age at death. Those with "reported" age at death number over 3,500 and were acquired from respondents to advertisements placed in relevant journals requesting information on individuals dying in their ninth decade or above.[1]

Table 1: Datasets in the "Maximal Length of Life" database

Dataset	Number in dataset	Number with death age	% with death age	Average entry age	Date of entry
English and Welsh Priests	4115	3523	85.6	27.5	1558-1800
British Members of Parliament	21161	15933	75.3	34.4	1529-1885
Rugby Old Boys	11287	6913	61.2	12.9	1675-1890
Scottish Ministers	9220	3144	34.0	35.5	1547-1914
Nuns	11982	9570	79.9	26.5	1581-1991
Advert Replies	3557	3557	100.0	-	C16th-C20th
TOTAL WITH AGE AT DEATH (excluding adverts)	**39083**				
TOTAL WITH AGE AT DEATH DYING BEFORE 1800	**14558**				

There are over 39,000 individuals in the database with "calculated" age at death data. These people derive from a number of secondary sources containing potted biographies of sub-groups of the British population from the sixteenth century

---

[1] The advertisement was placed in journals such as *Family Tree Magazine, The Genealogists Magazine, Local Population Studies* and *Family News and Digest Magazine.*

onwards. Those included are English and Welsh Catholic priests 1558 to 1800 (Bellenger 1884), British Members of Parliament from 1558 to 1885 (History of Parliament Trust), "old boys" of Rugby School from 1675 to 1890 (Solly 1933, Salt 1952), Scottish Ministers from 1558 to the nineteenth century (Scott 1915), and nuns from the sixteenth to the twentieth centuries[2]. The bias of the database towards the privileged and educated is an asset because these individuals are more likely than the general population to be documented in records other than parish registers and therefore aid the verification process.

a) "Reported" age at death dataset

Of the 3557 individuals who were reported to have reached age eighty or above, 89 were stated as centenarians of whom 21 were reported to have died before 1800. It is important to note the relative scarcity of reported centenarians considering the prevailing view that there has always been a wish to exaggerate age among the elderly. It is equally interesting that of those responses to the advertisements reporting a centenarian dying before 1800 and subsequently co-operating with the request for further information on the individuals, only 3 of the original 21 appear possibly verifiable. Several informants admitted that their original letter contained incorrect date information, others had gleaned their material from tombstones or burial registers and could find no additional supporting evidence whilst several had been given the information concerning the reported centenarian from a third party and so were of no further help.

The material on the three possibly genuine reported centenarians, Dorothy Jones (nee Williams), Elizabeth Edward(e)s (nee Owens) and John Lunniss, was acquired from two respondents, one of whom provided the information on the two women who were born in the same parish in the county of Clwyd at a similar point in time. Although the information regarding the two ladies is fairly convincing, it is perplexing that they both died paupers in the same township at a similar point in time; the chances of this happening are, to say the least, small.

---

[2]Database provided by Mr. M. Gandy and Mr. A. Nye

b) "Calculated" age at death datasets

Of the 39,083 individuals with "calculated" age at death information, 14,558 died before 1800. Among these individuals, 5 possible centenarians dying before 1800 were located:
i) Nuns Dame Gertrude Chillton and Dame Margaret Markhame
ii) Scottish Minister John Buchanan
iii) Member of Parliament William Badger
iv) English Catholic Priest Ferdinand Ashmall

In total there were 8 potential centenarians dying before 1800 in the *"Maximal Length of Life"* database. This might be deemed unrealistic in such a small population, despite the majority of the universe being selective as most were privileged and had survived infancy and childhood because the mean age at entry for the datasets was below twenty only for Rugby School old boys. How many, if any, of these preliminary claims of extreme longevity can be substantiated after the facts have been presented?

Before these individuals are discussed, in an attempt to reduce the "cult of centenarians" and to identify a definite maximal length of life in England before 1800 upon which we can build, attention should be paid to verifying those dying aged 97, 98 and 99 years old in the *"Maximal Length of Life"* database. At least one record appears to be watertight. Sir John Holland was born October 1603, matriculated fellow-commoner from Christs College Cambridge in March 1620/1 and was admitted to The Middle Temple 7 February 1622-23. He was a Member of Parliament between 1640 and 1679 and continued to hold local public offices until his death 19 January 1701, aged 98 years. This man's record and career is indisputable and lends weight to those supporting the claims of certain centenarians dying before 1800 because if individuals certainly lived into the latter part of the tenth decade of their life, it is highly likely that a number of others lived beyond this age.

Eight centenarians - fact or fiction?

As the evidence supporting each potential centenarian is detailed in turn, it will become clear, as discussed above, that the process of verification might be an impossible task. Problems met when undertaking the challenge are outlined and are as informative as the evidence gathered.

1. The three "reported" centenarians

a) *John Lunniss*

The case of John Lunniss was reported by a descendant. He states in one letter, *"Although, as I have learnt from my studies with the Open University, many facts in research cannot be proved with absolute certainty, I am confident that John the Younger was a centenarian"*. This statement, although a personal comment, is based upon the conclusion arrived at after the facts were analysed.

John Lunniss (Lonyes) was the son of Thomas Lonyes (Juror of Manor Court Shepreth 1540-1543; will made 20/04/1558; buried at Shepreth 1558) and Denyce (buried Shepreth 1560). There were 6 children in the family, John the Elder, Alice, Thomas, John the Younger (the reported centenarian), Edware and Katherine. As John the Elder died without issue in 1585, one of the chief beneficiaries of his will was his brother, John the Younger who inherited the original holding.

Thomas, a brother of John the Younger married Margaret and had a son named John who was baptized at Shepreth parish church of All Saints on 15 August 1567. This nephew of the reported centenarian died one year before John the Younger and he cannot be mistaken for his uncle because in his will the nephew left legacies for his children when they would reach the age of 21. John the Younger was buried at Shepreth on 27 June 1621 with a Latin insert in the burial register stating "of 107 years or thereabouts".

The parish register does not record any other ages at death, so the incumbent was obviously aware that he was dealing with special circumstances, whilst it is clear that the reported death date cannot be mixed up with a younger name-sake.

Unfortunately, there can only be an estimated date of birth as no records survive with this information. In addition, this man is followed through his life course by the use of indirect evidence from wills and parish register material which is less satisfactory than acquiring direct data. Hence, although there are no known name-sakes competing with the potential centenarian there is too little evidence to conclude this man was a centenarian at his death.

b) *Dorothy Jones (nee Williams)*

Dorothy Jones, both common names in this part of Wales, was reported to be a centenarian at her death in 1769 by a respondent to one of the advertisements. This lady is reported to have been baptized 14 September 1662 in the parish of Gresford in Clwyd. She married Humphre Jones of Llay on 7 January 1703 and after spending some time in the parish almshouse she was buried on 5 November 1769 with the parish burial register recording her age at death to be 106 years.

The late marriage of this lady is suggestive of an incorrect baptismal date. However, such marriages are reported by local historians to be common in this locale and the fact that the couple remained childless might support the claim of Dorothy's "calculated" late age of marriage.

A Dorothy Jones of Burton township (Gresford Parish) received payments from 1735 to 1743 from the overseer for keeping Cooper's boy and then received an allowance from 1744 to 1769 when the burial register suggests she died. A grave in the churchyard states *"Underneath lies the body of Dorothy Jones of Gresford who departed this life the 1st day of November 1769 aged 106 years"*.

There are name-sakes in the parish registers, but only two could feasibly be mistaken for this lady. A (.....) Williams, daughter of John of Burton, was born 25 December 1672, which would make her aged thirty if she is the person who married Humphre Jones of Llay on 7 January 1703; perhaps more realistic than the reported baptismal date given for Dorothy Williams? However, if the marriage and death date belonged to this baptismal date, the age at death would still be 97. The other option is the burial record of the Dorothy Jones of Llay (Gresford parish) who was buried 7 June 1729. It is possible that upon marriage Dorothy migrated to Llay with her husband and died there in 1729.

Although the burial register notation and the gravestone information point to this woman being the same female who was baptized in Gresford 14 September 1662, the two alternatives outlined above introduce an element of uncertainty. It is the second option which is of most concern because this would make her under seventy years of age at her death, whereas the first would place above ninetyfive.

c)   *Elizabeth Edward(e)s (nee Owens)*

The case of Elizabeth Edward(e)s, again not uncommon names in this part of Wales, reported by the respondent who informed us of Dorothy Williams, has even less supporting evidence than the afore mentioned.

Elizabeth is reported to have been baptized in Burton (Gresford parish) on 1 March 1678/9, to have married Thomas Edwardes 6 October 1695 and to have been buried as a pauper aged 104 on 26 January 1783 as Elizabeth Edwards of Mold Parish. Additional evidence includes the recording from the paupers' weekly allowance for the poor of Mold of Elizabeth Edward(e)s receiving funds. However, a gravestone does not survive and the burial register states that Elizabeth was of Mold Parish whilst the other vital events state that she was of Burton in the parish of Gresford. Did she migrate to Mold at some point and return to her roots to enter the almshouse towards the end of her life or does the burial record belong to a namesake?

Unfortunately, there is not enough evidence to rigorously support any of the three claims of centenarian outlined above. Dorothy Williams is the most promising case but there is still enough doubt for the sceptics to remain unimpressed that any of the above three were undoubtedly centenarians at their death. The fact that all three had common names with close relatives of other generations being namesakes helps to complicate the situation. Yet many of the namesakes can be ruled out of contention for the vital events allotted to the reported centenarian.

Unfortunately, as in the instance of Dorothy Williams, it only takes one of the vital events allotted to the centenarian to be challenged by one alternative to make the identification problematic. The lack of information in years between vital events is of concern for three people with common names because doubt of correct linkage can be placed on the reported baptismal, marriage and burial dates.

2. The five "calculated" centenarians

a) *Dame Gertrude Chillton (nun)*

Henrietta Chillton was the daughter of Christopher Chillton of Newcastle, Northumberland. She was received into the Brussels convent of the Benedictine nuns 7 September 1689 and was invested with the holy habit, taking the religious name of Gertrude on 5 April 1693. She was professed 3 June 1694 at the age of 19 and died in 1794.

The above information is provided in the annals of the order to which Dame Gertrude Chillton belonged. Unfortunately, no record can be found of either her birth or death date as few English Catholic records survive from this period. It is likely that the reported year of death, 1794, is incorrect because if it were to be accurate she would have been 119 years old at her death. It is more likely that she departed this life in 1694 at a young age. As there is absolutely no supporting evidence, little progress can be made in the attempt to verify the report of this individual, firstly because few English Catholic records survive from before the nineteenth century and secondly because this lady's adult life was spent abroad, finding further evidence is virtually an impossible, and certainly an impractical task.

b) *Dame Margaret Markhame*

Margaret was the daughter of George Markhame Esquire of Ollerton, Sherwood Forest in Nottinghamshire. Like her father, Margaret's mother, Judith Witherwick Fitzwilliams, was also from a wealthy landed family. At least one of Margaret's brothers, after his training at Douai, joined her in devoting his life to God. Dame Margaret professed with the English Benedictine nuns on 27 December 1639 at the age of 22 years. In 1652 she was sent to Boulogne and later to Pontoise, before visiting Ireland in 1687. Her obituary states that she died in the 105th year of her life and the 77th of her profession on 25 July 1717. However, if she was aged 22 when she professed in 1639 she would be aged 99 or 100 at her death.

There are several points to be made about the verification of the age at death of this nun. Although a birth record has not been found, the stated age at profession is probably reliable. Her career, situation and age at death are detailed and convincing. However, like other obituary notices which both date and specify the age at profession and date of death, the stated age at death often deviates from that calculated. Although no evidence has been found to support the information provided in the obituary notice, unlike that of Dame Gertrude Chillton, it was a detailed and continuous record of her adult life as a nun. Consequently, there is sufficient evidence to argue that the date of and age at profession, and date of death are accurate, making this lady at least 99 years of age at the end of her life.

c) *John Buchanan (Scottish Minister)*

The publication, *Fasti Ecclesiae Scoticanae* (Scott 1915) states that John Buchanan was born in 1619, son of John Buchanan, a merchant in Stirling. He was ordained on 29 April 1691 and he died 27 February 1726. He married Catherine Spruell and had a son John who was baptized 20 December 1694 and who was his successor as the minister of Covington Parish, Stirlingshire.

The birth date of John Buchanan of 1619 should be treated with great suspicion because if it is correct, he would have been aged 72 when he was ordained, aged 75 at the birth of his namesake and aged 107 at his death. His age at ordination and at the birth of his son although not impossible according to experts on Scottish history, is highly improbable. There was possibly a typing error in the birth date but this cannot be confirmed because his birth record cannot be located and is not in The International Genealogical Index. Consequently, in the absence of any other corroborating evidence, there is reason for scepticism about this individual having been a centenarian at death.

d) *William Badger (Member of Parliament)*

In the publication edited by Hasler (1981) titled *The Commons 1558-1603*, a potted biography is given of the Member of Parliament for Winchester in 1597, a William Badger. It provides an approximate date of birth of c1523 based on the date by which he was a freeman, 1551. The biography states that he was an attorney, three times mayor of Winchester in 1572, 1586 and 1597 respectively and the Member of Parliament for Winchester in 1597 when aged about seventy. He died intestate and was buried in Winchester Cathedral 18 January 1629. The biography further states, *"Though it is stretching credulity to have a man make his first appearance in Parliament aged over seventy and live to be a centenarian, the evidence in Badger's case seems conclusive, both as regards its known dates and the absence of any break in career which might imply confusion between name-sakes"* (Vol.1 p.383). It is clear that he had two sons and one daughter, one son was named Robert and the other William. A birth record is available for Robert but not for William (junior) or Grace, the daughter. However, William (junior) can be identified as entering Winchester School in 1561 aged ten years, going up to New College Oxford in 1569 and becoming a fellow there 1571-74. Between 1575 and 1576 William Badger (junior) was admitted to Lincoln's Inn before being presented by William Badger (senior) to the prebendary of Beaminster Secunda. Hence, William (senior) must have been born about 1523 as stated in the International Genealogical Index. In the surviving manuscripts for Winchester it states that William Badger the three times mayor of Winchester became a Member of Parliament in 1597. However, it makes no comment on the individual's age which could imply that the individual was not deemed aged or unusual in any way and that he was known to the community. If it had been William (junior) who was elected, it is likely his relationship to his locally renowned father, William (senior) the three times mayor of the city, would have been commented upon.

Hence, although the information is not conclusive and might be slightly confusing, there is a fairly solid case that the Member of Parliament for Winchester in 1597 died a centenarian in 1627, having had his son Robert in c1550 and William shortly after, and having held a series of public offices from the middle of the sixteenth century until his old age. The fact that his precise birth date is unknown does not disqualify this individual because supporting evidence suggests his date of birth to within a short time span.

e) *Ferdinand Ashmall (secular Catholic priest)*

The case for Ferdinand Ashmall dying a centenarian is strong and surprising because research has shown that married women had a higher survival rate than unmarried men. Luckily, because his family was of some social standing they were "visible" in documents and their pedigree has been detailed.

Ferdinand was born at Amerston in County Durham on 9 January 1695. His father Thomas and his mother Mary Addison bought an estate at Amerston which became the family seat for several years. Ferdinand was admitted to Lisbon College (Portugal) on 9 August 1711 at the age of fifteen to train for the priesthood. He was ordained 18 February 1720 and returned to England in 1723, becoming the chaplain to Mary Salvin at Old Elvet, County Durham, for the next four years until her death. In 1727 Ferdinand retired to his father's estate at Amerston to recover from ill health. Nothing is known of his activities until 1745 when he became priest at New House near Esh, County Durham, where he remained until his death on 5 February 1798 aged 104 years. His will had been made on 14 April 1787 and was proved on 10 February 1798, leaving his money and goods to his niece and the children of his brother-in-law. His obituary in *The Gentleman's Magazine* states, *"At Newhouse, near Esh, County Durham, in the 104th year of his age, and the 73rd of his ministry, the Reverend Ferdinand Ashmall, a Roman Catholic clergyman"*. In Buller's Record and Recollections of St. Cuthbert's College, Ushaw, it states that *the ancient and venerable priest, the Reverend Ferdinando Ashmall, who had charge for so many years of the (R.C.) mission at Newhouse, died on February 5th 1798, aged 104 and "was buried at Esh, in the graveyard of the Protestant Chapel"*. Additional information about this incumbent includes the inheritance of his father's estate in 1758 after the death of his two brothers Thomas and Robert. He was listed in the *Returns of Papists 1767* as Mr. Ashmon, priest of Esh Chapelry, aged 70 and resident for twenty three years whilst *Laity's Directory* for 1799 records him in the obituary notices as dying in February 1798, R. Ferdinand Ashmall, Durham, age 104.

This man could have been mistaken for only one known name-sake, his uncle. This older Ferdinand Ashmall was also a priest whose life course can be verified as being independent of that of his nephew, and so avoiding confusion between the two relations. The author of the book *English and Welsh Priests 1558-1800* (Bellinger 1884) in which all priests associated with this geographical area are listed and details given, states in a letter about this potential centenarian, *"His name-sake Ferdinand Ashmall (born 1650) definitely died in 1712. Thus the man retired to Amerston was almost certainly the long-lived Ferdinand Ashmall ....The ordination lists of the English College giving Ferdinand Ashmall as of Lisbon College and ordained in 1723 are complete. It is unlikely anyone of this name would be ordained from an Irish College....In this case longevity is more likely than imposture".*

Long Livers in the "Maximal Length of Life Database"

There is little doubt that many potential centenarians from the past will never be proved or disproved purely because of the lack of surviving records providing definite evidence. Researching certain types of people makes the task more difficult as, for instance, the survival rate of non-conformist vital event records is lower than for conformists before 1800 in England and Wales and those who were neither rich nor poor tend to be less "visible" as they were less regularly recorded than those at extreme ends of the social and economic spectrum. On the other hand, researching males of the conformist persuasion who spent most of their life in England and who held some sort of official position is an advantage because in their case evidence is more likely to be available.

The eight examples discussed above exhibit a range of difficulties which might be impossible to overcome, forcing a negative conclusion to the search for verification. The stumbling block for Dorothy Jones (nee Williams) was an alternative date of death which cannot be proven not to belong to the lady in question because upon marriage it is possible that she moved to her husband's abode in Llay. In the case of Elizabeth Edward(e)s (nee Owens) the main obstacle was the lack of supporting evidence linking the vital events, the poor law register and ultimately the burial record to the same woman. The case of Dame Gertrude Chillton is the same but complicated by her adulthood having been spent overseas. The major concern in the instance of the Scottish Minister is possible incorrect typing in his potted biography of his birth date resulting in a rather late age at ordination and the birth of his namesake. Finally, in the case of the Member of Parliament William Badger, there is a suggestion that there is confusion between himself and his son.

Conclusion

a) General

The results of this study certainly suggest that some persons did survive to become centenarians in the high mortality regime of the pre-demographic transition era and the problems with historical research which have been highlighted during this study have failed to force a negative conclusion. Despite the imperfect evidence, the nun Dame Margaret Markhame, the Member of Parliament William Badger and Catholic priest Ferdinand Ashmall may be seen as very promising cases of examples of centenarians dying before 1800. In addition, there are others who died aged just under the "magic" figure of one hundred.

It is important to remember that although expectation of life at birth was low before 1800 in England and Wales, if one survived into young adulthood one could on average expect to live into the sixth or seventh decade. Although mortality after this age was high and stable, there is no reason to believe that small numbers could not live on into their eleventh decade. The evidence supports this theory.

b) *Implications*

The implications are two-fold. Firstly, although statistical modelling indicates that the probability of surviving to the age of 100 before 1800 was small, this study argues that such extreme long livers did exist. If mortality in old age was high but stable for at least the three centuries leading up to 1800, then it is feasible that there were centenarians long before the beginning of the nineteenth century. Historians should not be dissuaded from pursuing information supporting the claims of long-lived individuals and believing them to be true centenarians after persuasive evidence has been presented simply because statistically, it is highly improbable that the individual found was a centenarian at death.

The results of this study may also imply that the maximal length of life in the high mortality era was not significantly lower than today. If Reverend Ferdinand Ashmall really was 104 years old at his death and William Badger died at a similar age, there was likely to have been someone dying at a later age in the population at risk of 22 to 25 million in England between 1537 and 1800. The search for such a person must continue because he or she has not yet been located due to the problems associated with the verification of centenarians in a historical setting. On the other hand, the oldest ever verified person is the French super-centenarian Madame Calment who is presently 120 years old. There is unlikely to have been another person living to above this age in recent times because the developed registration systems throughout the world would have identified such a spectacularly long-lived person.

Perhaps the evidence suggests that rather than absolute change with the shift in mortality there has been some form of continuity in observed maximal length of life over a long period of time and less change in the last two centuries than at earlier points in the life cycle, including old age. Parkin (1992) summarises this argument when he implies that there has indeed been more continuity than change, stating *"...despite the "demographic transition" and the advances in medicine this century, a person does not live significantly longer today than his or her ancestor did in the historical past. The simple fact is that more people survive into old age today, not that they live any longer than elderly people in past times"*. However, more evidence concerning maximal length of life in the high mortality past must be presented before this argument can be pursued further. Approaching this task by attempting to verify literary evidence detailing reported centenarians in the past might be a useful exercise.

Literature

Bailey, T. 1857. Records of Longevity: with an Introductory Discourse on Vital Statistics. *Darton & Co.*, London.

Bellenger, A. 1884. English and Welsh Priests 1558-1800. *Downside Abbey.*

Ernest, M. 1938. The Longer Life. *Adam & Co.*, London.

Hasler, P.W.(Ed.). 1981. The House of Commons 1558-1603. *Her Majesty's Stationary Office*, London.

History of Parliament Trust. The History of Parliament. 21 volumes published by the History of Parliament Trust containing potted biographies for all Members of Parliament between 1439 and 1975.

Kannisto, V. 1988. On the Survival of Centenarians and the Span of Life. *Population Studies No. 42.*

Kannisto, V., J. Lauritsen, A.R. Thatcher and J.W. Vaupel. 1993. Reductions in Mortality at Advanced Ages. *Population Studies of Aging #4*, Centre for Health and Social Policy, Odense University.

Parkin, T. 1992. Demography and Roman Society. *The John Hopkins University Press.*

Salt, F.J. 1952. Rugby School Register 1858-1891: Revised. *George Over Ltd.*

Scott, H. 1915. Fasti Ecclesiae Scoticanae. *Oliver and Boyd*, Edinburgh.

Solly, G. 1933. Rugby School Register: Annotated Vol. 1 1675-1857. *George Over Ltd.*

Thoms, W.J. 1873. Human Longevity. Its Facts and its Fictions. *John Murray*, London.

Thoms, W.J. 1879. The Longevity of Man. *Frederic Norgate*, London.

Weber, H. 1914. On Means for the Prolongation of Life. 4th ed. *J. Bale & Co.*, London.

Wrigley, E.A., and R.S. Schofield. 1981. The Population History of England, 1541-1871. *Harvard University Press.*

Record Longevity in Chinese History - Evidence from the Wang Genealogy

by Zhongwei Zhao

Records of extreme human longevity are frequently found in many countries. Some of them suggest that in the remote past there were people who lived to very old ages, or even became centenarians. Yet questions such as to what extent these records can be accepted as historically accurate; what was the highest age that was ever reached by a human individual in the past; was there any person who indeed became a centenarian before the 19th century; and when did the human lifespan first break the one hundred year record in the world still need to be adequately examined. Some scholars, working on historical records in a number of western countries, have recently proposed that there was in fact no centenarian before 1800 (Jeune, this monograph). Could this suggestion be true of the population of the world as a whole? This chapter, by presenting a theoretical model and some empirical evidence, attempts to further improve our knowledge on these questions.

The longest human lifespan recorded, mortality level and population size - a model

What is the biological limit of the human lifespan or whether such a limit indeed exists are questions under investigation. However, if we assume that there is such a limit but it is still far away for the human population to reach - say the limit is 150 years - then in a homogeneous population where the risk of death is the same for everyone at birth and how long a person can live is mainly affected by what he or she experiences after birth, the occurrence of centenarians, or the number of people who could reach extremely old ages, would be primarily associated with two factors: mortality level and population size. The first determines at what speed a population of a birth cohort would die out, and the second determines, under a particular mortality level, the actual number of people in that cohort who could have reached a certain age. If we also assume that mortality in human population more or less follows the Gompertz law,[1] the relationship can be illustrated by the graphs in Figure 1.

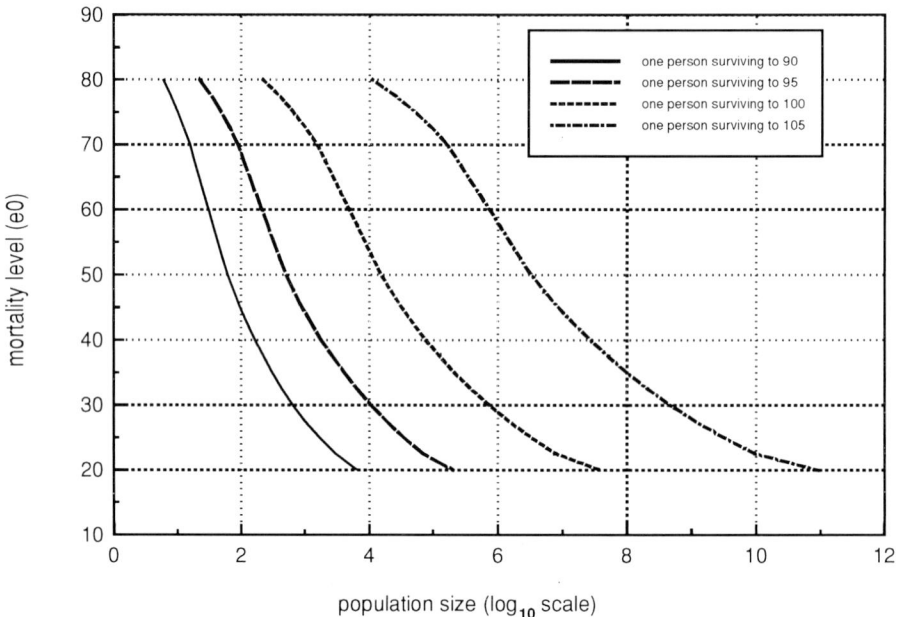

Figure 1

The curves in Figure 1 are based on Coale-Demeny family of model life tables, Region west, Females. The number of people who could survive to very old ages has been recalculated by using the Gompertz formula given by Coale and Demeny in

---

[1] Benjamin Gompertz suggested that mortality rates increase exponentially at old ages. This suggestion has been referred as the Gompertz law. Whether mortality change among very old people follows this law is a question which is under debate and is being empirically tested. Recently, studies show that this law may not be universally applicable to all species and some even suggest that in some human populations mortality at very old ages may not exponentially increase but level off or decrease after a certain point. However, because the major focus here is whether centenarians could exist at all in the past rather than what law was precisely followed by human mortality, the Gompertz law has been used to produce a theoretical value of the number of very old people which may be achieved under the given mortality level. This value would be the low limit, if mortality does not accelerate exponentially at very old ages but stabilizes at a certain level or slows down. For further discussion, see Gompertz 1825, Barinaga 1991, 1992, Thatcher 1992, Carey et al 1992.

order to get more accurate results.² In this figure, the Y axis represents mortality level and is labeled by its outcome - life expectancy at birth. The X axis indicates population size and the $\log_{10}$ scale is used to resolve the difficulty in mapping numbers with huge discrepancies. The curves show the size of a population of a birth cohort which, under the given age specific mortality rates indicated by the level of life expectancy at birth, could produce one person surviving to age 90, 95, 100, and 105. These curves also show how the number of people who could reach very old ages would change in relation to changes in mortality level and population size.³

The curve representing one person surviving to age 100, for example, suggests that under the mortality level which gives a life expectation at birth of 20 years, out of a birth cohort of about 40 million people perhaps only one person could survive to age 100. When the mortality declines and the life expectancy at birth rises to 30 years, the size of the birth cohort which could possibly produce a centenarian will decrease to about a million. If these curves are taken as roughly representing the surviving experiences of the human population in the past, then the following observations could be made in relation to our understanding of the recent rapid increase in the number of very old people in the world.

First, the number of people who could reach very old ages is negatively related to mortality level, and positively related to life expectancy at birth. The lower the mortality, the smaller the number of people from which a centenarian could emerge. If a population experiences a force of mortality which gives a life expectancy at birth of 55 years, for example, in a birth cohort of 10 thousand people, only about one person could reach age 100. While under the mortality which gives a life expectancy of 80 years, the size of the birth cohort which is likely to produce a centenarian may be reduced to less than three hundred. In other words, if population size remains unchanged, falling mortality or increasing life expectancy will lead to a greater

---

² The formula is expressed as $l_x = l_{80} \, exp \, [-(u(80) \, / \, k) \, (e^{k(x-80)}-1)]$ and is provided in Coale and Demeny (1983 p.20). It should be noted that another formula which they presented for calculating "k" and set out in the same page contains a mistake. The formula should be written as $k = log \, (u(105) \, / \, u(77.5)) \, / \, 27.5$, or $k = (log \, u(105) - log \, u(77.5)) \, / \, 27.5$, instead of $k = log \, (u(105) - u(77.5)) \, / \, 27.5$.

³ These curves suggest that if a population of a birth cohort of a certain size went through a set of age specific mortality rates, which are represented by life expectation at birth in the figure, then among them one person would reach a particular age. It should be aware that the theoretical value of this kind is different from that which could be observed in an actual population where mortality levels have not been constant and the occurrence of centenarians or those surviving to very old people is also affected by many other factors. Nevertheless, such a value can been seen as an average which is likely to be found if demographic conditions similar to our assumptions indeed exist.

number of octogenarians, nonagenarians and centenarians.

Second, the number of people who could reach very old ages is positively related to population size. This not only means that when population size increases N times, the number of those who could survive to a certain age will also increase about N times, but also that those who could reach extremely old ages are much more likely to be found in large populations. Under a mortality level which gives a life expectancy at birth of 20 years, for instance, if a birth cohort consists of 200 thousand people, then there may be only one person who could possibly survive to age 95 and it will be exceedingly unlikely that any person will reach age 100. If the population size increases for 200 times (from 200 thousand to 40 million), however, the number of people who could survive to age 95 will rise to about 200, and among them, some may be able to live to 98 or 99, and centenarians are also likely to emerge.

Third, the ratio between the number of people reaching age X and those reaching age X+N is not a constant. It changes considerably in responding to a change in mortality level. According to the graph, for example, when average life expectancy at birth is 20 years, among some 200 people who reach age 95 there may be only one person who could survive to age 100. In contrast, when life expectancy at birth rises to 80 years, one in twenty of those reaching age 95 may live to age 100. Although these statistics, which are derived from the model life tables, may not accurately represent the experience of any population, the trend indicated by them is in agreement with the findings of recent empirical research (Kannisto 1988, Thatcher 1992, Vaupel and Lundström 1993).

The above analysis seems to be helpful in answering the questions set out at the beginning of this chapter. Some scholars have claimed that there might have been no true centenarian before the 19th century or before the onset of industrialization. Such a suggestion is likely to be true, if it is applied to only the populations studied by them, because most of the historical populations which have so far been investigated were in fact relatively small in size and in these populations mortality was fairly high before the nineteenth century. Under such circumstances, centenarians would be extremely difficult to find. Yet, if we increase the size of the population being studied or choose populations with relatively low mortality, the above conclusion may not hold. Indeed, the research on Chinese genealogies which will be reported in the following suggests that in China some people might have become centenarians well before the year 1800, although their number must always have been exceedingly small in the past even in that large country.

Data source - the Wang Genealogy

Differing from in most western countries where parish registers made in the last few centuries are widely available and have consequently become the major source of historical demography, in China thousands of family or lineage genealogies exist and they provide the most important data source for the study of Chinese population history.

The records concerning the longest human lifespan reported in the next section are taken from the General Genealogy of Wang (Wang Shi Tong Pu). Wang is the surname of those recorded in the genealogy. This genealogy consists of 106 volumes. The first generation in the genealogy, according to the records, lived around 500 BC, and some of those who lived at the end of the last century were listed as the descendants in the eighty-ninth generation. Altogether, around 30,000 people were recorded.

In the Wang Genealogy, personal information was given for each male individual. These records were arranged by generations and by family or lineage branches. People of the same branch were normally descended from a common ancestor and lived in the same area. Initially, these genealogical records were kept by each particular family or lineage. During the second half of the last century, they were collected together and edited by a person named Wang Yongjing and his sons. The records used in this study were published at the end of the 19th century.

The social status of those who were recorded in the genealogy was relatively high. This was particularly the case for those who lived in the very early period. It may be said that before the year 1000 AD, the recorded people largely belonged to upper and upper middle classes. Thereafter, the component of those from middle, or perhaps lower, class increased. Nevertheless, people who came from upper middle, or upper, class still made up a substantial part. For these reasons, the social demographic phenomena found in this population may not represent those which might be observed in the Chinese population as a whole.

Because the Wang Genealogy covered a very long period, consisted of a great number of people, and was originally produced by various families and lineages according to different rules, the information recorded varied considerably from entry to entry. A detailed record normally included the name of the given person, the generation to which he belonged, order of birth, name of his father, precise dates of birth and death, age at death, number of wives (specified as first wife, second wife and concubines), number of sons and daughters (their mothers sometimes being specified), wife's age at death (occasionally with date), and political and academic achievements.

Most records, however, are not complete and the information provided by them is rather limited. A considerable number of entries contain only name, generation, name of father, and number of sons. This is particularly the case for records made for people who lived in the very early period. Moreover, under-registration of various kinds also existed. Apart from the fact that most women were excluded from the genealogy, two types of persons were apparently under-recorded: those who died young, particularly those who died at very young ages; and those whose information could not be traced. The second type of omission was occasionally noted in the genealogy by "Wu Kao" - not traceable.[4]

Two general observations can be made about the Wang Genealogy. Firstly, historical records which cover such a long period have never been found in other countries. Even in China, records of this kind are exceedingly rare. This makes the Wang Genealogy very valuable in the study of social demographic history. Secondly, because of various kinds of under-registration, we will probably never know how many people were omitted from the Wang Genealogy, or the size of the population from which these recorded people came. This limits the usefulness of the Wang Genealogy considerably.

Recorded maximum human lifespan in the Wang Genealogy

In the Wang Genealogy, those who died young (under age 25), especially those who died very young, are apparently under-recorded. Because of that, we are not in a position to investigate infant and child mortality. However, the data analysis suggests that mortality patterns among those who died between age 30 and 75 are similar to those indicated by Coale-Demeny model life table, East region, Level 7 or 8, Males. Among those who were recorded as surviving to 80 and over, the mortality rate calculated from the genealogical records is likely to be lower than what actually existed in this lineage population. This is mainly due to the fact that in the genealogy people who died at very old ages tended to be over represented. Since our major focus is recorded maximum lifespan rather than mortality patterns as such, these

---

[4] In most Chinese genealogies, there are no individual records for women, although they may be mentioned as wives in the records of their husbands, or as daughters in the records of their fathers. For discussion of under-registration of other kinds, see Zhao (1994).

details are not discussed here.⁵

The limitation imposed by various types of under-registration is apparent. Because of the selective bias which is created by these problems, we should be very cautious whenever we try to use the findings derived from such a sample to generalize the situation of the entire population. Nevertheless, these problems do not prevent us from describing the character of the sample itself. Although the over-representation of those with longer lifespan tends to make the age specific mortality rates less reliable, it has no serious impact on our searching for the maximum length of lifespan reached by human populations in the past, if the recorded ages in the genealogy are accurate.⁶

In the Wang Genealogy, dates of birth and death are available for some 2,500 males, and they show a very high degree of consistency with recorded ages at death. Since these records are ostensibly more reliable than others, they have been used as the major data source in this study. Among these 2,500 males, about two hundred were born before the year 1000, some one thousand between the year 1000 and 1500, the remaining thousand being born after the 15th century.

In this study, the traditional Chinese calendar year has been converted into the modern calendar year and the age of every person has been calculated in the conventional way.⁷ There were 209 of the sample of nearly 2,500 men who were recorded to have survived to age 80 and over. Half of these 209 lived before 1500, and half of them after that date. Of the 209 men, 22 died between 90 and 94, six between 95 and 99, and one died at age 102 in the year 1513.

Those who survived for more than 95 years are listed in Table 1. Three of the males died at age 96. One of them was born in the 13th century and the other two in the 15th century. There were also three who were reported to have reached age

---

⁵ A detailed discussion of mortality patterns in this lineage population is presented in Zhao (1994).

⁶ Indeed, under the condition that the recorded ages are accurate and reliable, this disadvantage can even be seen as an advantage. According to figure 1, for example, under a high mortality regime, a population of millions might produce only a small number of nonagenarians and possibly a couple of rare centenarians. Yet, detailed personal records of a population with such a size are not available for any population living before 1750. Even if such data are available, data input and analysis may be very time consuming. In this sense, the selection by the genealogy compiler of those who died at very advanced ages saves us an enormous amount of work.

⁷ In the genealogy, age at death was counted in the traditional Chinese way - i.e. when a person was born he or she was counted as one year old. In this paper, however, a person's age have been computed by subtracting the date of birth from the date of death.

Table 1. Males aged 95 and over in Wang Genealogy

Name	Year of birth	Year of death	Age at death
Tiansheng	1161	1258	97
Qian	1202	1298	96
Yi	1237	1335	98
Xinglian	1411	1513	102
Yu	1452	1548	96
Shizhong	1484	1580	96
Yanzhen	1598	1697	99

97, 98 and 99, and were born in the 12th, 13th and 16th centuries respectively. The one male centenarian lived between 1411 and 1513.[8] In addition, there were also six old women who were recorded to have survived to age 95 and over, and are listed in table 2. They were aged 95, 96, 97 (two persons), 100, and 103, and were born in the 17th, 16th, 15th, 17th, 16th and 13th centuries respectively. Most of these old people, especially these old women, are found in the families or lineages where genealogical records of higher quality were kept. Because there are no individual entries for females in the Wang Genealogy, no dates of birth and dates of death can be used to check the reliability of these reported ages. However, other information may be brought up as reference. For the lady who was recorded to have reached age 100 in the 17th century, for instance, the genealogy recorded that by order of the imperial government an archway was built in front of her house and she was given a title to honour her very impressive success in archiving great longevity.

According to these records, therefore, centenarians already existed in China at a period as early as the 13th century. Mortality was high in Chinese history, and it was considerably higher than that recorded in European countries at least during the last one or two hundred years. But China had and still has the largest population in the world. Research suggests that the Chinese population had already reached one hundred million by the 11th century, and hundreds of millions of Chinese people lived and died during the last thousand years. In addition to the Wangs, there were

---

[8] In the Wang Genealogy, there were also several other males who were reported to have become centenarians, but because their dates of birth and death are not available, these cases are not presented here.

Table 2. Females aged 95 and over in Wang Genealogy

Name of husband	Century of husband's death	Age at death	Husband's age at death
Wenrong	13	103	-
Lun	15	97	69
Yongguang	16	96	71
Shangmian	16	100	-
Xizan	17	95	-
Kequan	17	97	75

also hundreds of thousands of Lis, Zhangs, Lius, Yangs and many more people with other surnames. This huge population size over time may have given China the chance of producing the first few centenarians in the world history.

Furthermore, average mortality, as a combined result of low living standard, frequent famines, wars and diseases, was certainly high in Chinese history. But because of the better living standard which was enjoyed by the upper class, the long history of Chinese medicine, the prosperity of the early Chinese civilization and socio-economic development, the mortality experienced by certain social groups might not have been so excessive. Indeed, the mortality level prevalent among the Chinese elites could even have been lower than those found among their European counterparts.[9] The people recorded in the Wang genealogy were largely a collection of those who belonged to this social group, and some of them were likely to have reached very old ages. For these reasons, it is not impossible that a couple of centenarians could be found in China several hundred years ago.

Reliability of the recorded age

The above discussion inevitably leads to the question to what extent these longevity records can be accepted as historical facts, or to what extent the age records in the Wang Genealogy can be seen as reliable? Age exaggeration has been found in many populations and it has been particularly a problem among old people (Wilmoth and

---

[9] Analysis of the Wang Genealogy and results published by some other researchers indicate that before the mid-18th century, mortality among some Chinese elite groups might be very close or even lower than those found among the European upper class (Zhao 1994).

Lundström 1995). It is true that in Chinese history there were always incentives for people to exaggerate their ages and old people were respected by the society. But, disincentives were there as well, and the punishment for exaggerating age could be severe. In the Wang Genealogy, recording people's ages at death seems not to have been affected by these factors, and there was no observable fraud.[10]

Admittedly, dates of birth and death are not available for the majority in the Wang Genealogy. But this does not in itself mean that the recorded date of birth, date of death and age at death are unreliable. In Chinese history, detailed records of date and even hours of birth were made for each newborn in many families partly due to the fact that they believed that a person's fortune and destiny were largely determined by the time of his or her birth. Although the major users of these records, until recently, were not demographers but fortune tellers, the fortune tellers and those who asked about their destiny also treated the quality of these records quite seriously. Moreover, if the genealogy compilers had intended to falsify ages for those whose ages at death went unrecorded, the number of these people would be very small rather than large. Data analysis indicates that in spite of the problems caused by various kinds of under-registration, no obvious age heaping can be identified among those whose ages at death were given. Recorded dates of birth and death, and recorded ages of death show a very high degree of consistency.

Another circumstance indicating the reliability of the recorded ages is that in the Wang Genealogy, as in other Chinese genealogies, dates of birth and of death were registered according to the traditional Chinese calendar rather than modern calendar reckoning. This made it rather difficult for people to forge age for themselves and even more so for their ancestors.

Chinese history has been divided into some twenty dynasties since the "Xia" period (from about 2100 BC to about 1500 BC). Every dynasty, depending on the length of the time it lasted, was ruled by a number of emperors. Each of them, ascending the throne, would start a "new" period by issuing a new "Nian Hao" - the name of the period to be governed by the new imperial figure. The first year after such a "Nian Hao" began would be year one, and the second year two and so on. When the old ruler died or when the new one took over, the "Nian Hao" would normally be changed and the year would be counted from one again. In some

---

[10] According to the genealogy, for example, Wang Yongjing, the genealogy compiler, lived to age 54. During his lifetime, he married twice and took in four concubines. His first wife died at age 35. The four concubines died at age 20, 17, 23 and 42 respectively. The age at death of his second wife was not recorded and it was likely that she was still alive when the genealogy was published. Here, the genealogy compilers do not seem to have attempted to exaggerate the death ages for these people at all.

dynasties, an imperial ruler might announce several different "Nian Hao" during the period of his or her control.

In Chinese history, when the year was recorded, people would normally record both such a "Nian Hao" and the number of years since the given "Nian Hao" started. Some time the number of years was alternatively recorded according to the traditional "Sixty Sexagenary Cycle" method.[11] This means that counterfeiting ages for those who lived in the past could turn out to be a somewhat intricate task. In a society where the modern calendar is used, forging a death age and the date of death is a simple matter. All you need to do is simply to decide the date of birth, and then by adding the assumed age at death you will get the date of death. But under the traditional Chinese calendar reckoning system, forging an age at death may have required extensive knowledge of dynastic history and involve some fairly complicated calculations.

Given the above considerations, it seems reasonable to suggest that although many problems exist in the Wang Genealogy, in most cases recorded ages seem to be reliable, especially those where dates of birth and death are given.

Concluding remarks

Because of high mortality in the past and the under-registration problems which exist in Chinese genealogy data, suspicion about the reliability of these longevity records may exist. Although we should be cautious about the credibility of these records and further investigation should be carried out on other historical materials, it would be unwise to completely reject the suggestion that some people could survive to very old ages or even become centenarians in the past.

Some people tend to believe that mortality change has been a linear decline - mortality was higher in the past and is lower now, and the earlier the period, the higher the mortality. Because mortality was high in the past, the occurrence of centenarians would be impossible. This suggestion, however, may not be true. The work on the Wang Genealogy shows that over a period of nearly a thousand of years, long-term mortality patterns were fairly stable in the population being studied. Data provided by Liu also indicate that in a much larger lineage population, the mortality level might not have changed or only had some marginal changes from the 16th

---

[11] This method treats sixty years as a cycle and it uses a particular combination of two Chinese characters to name each year. The same combination of Chinese characters will be used again when a new cycle starts.

century to the 18th century, perhaps even to the early 20th century (see Liu 1992 and Zhao 1994). If this indeed is the case, then it would be justifiable to say that what we have found in an 18th century or a 19th century population could also be found in a 15th century or a 14th century population. Similarly, if people could reach an age of a hundred of years in the 18th or the 19th century, there would be no reason why they could not become centenarians in the earlier time, if the population size was large enough. Mortality was high in the past, and this certainly considerably constrained the chance of people surviving to very high ages. But the high mortality did not make it impossible. In this regard, the evidence found in the Qing Imperial Genealogy, which is now being investigated by James Lee and his colleagues, has provided an important reference.[12]

As far as the quality of and the detailed information provided by the data are concerned, the Qing Imperial Genealogy may be one of the best historical demographic data sets in the world and is certainly one of the best historical data sets in China. In this genealogy, 96 per cent of personal records contain a precise year, month or even day of death; and the proportion of those with precise date of birth are even higher. The records made for males are more complete and more accurate than those for females.

According to Lee and his colleagues, mortality in this population was very high, in spite of the fact that these people were the most privileged in the country. Life expectancy at birth was less than 25 years among those who were born between 1700 and 1720. It was lower than 30 years among those who were born between 1720 and 1750. The mortality experienced by the next eight (ten-year) birth cohorts was slightly lower than that experienced by their predecessors, but life expectancy at birth was still lower than 35 years for most of the birth cohorts. In other words, the life expectancy at birth recorded in these 13 (ten-year) birth cohorts varied between those indicated by Coale-Demeny model life tables, Region west, Level 3 and Level 9, but was never higher. Adult mortality in this population was very high. In these birth cohorts, for example, life expectancy at age 30 and 50 was noticeably lower than those set by the Model life tables, Region west, Level 5 (Lee et al 1994). However, among those recorded people, a couple of centenarians have been found. According

---

[12] Soon after the Qing replaced the Ming in 1644, the Office of the Imperial Lineage was established (in 1652) to register lineage members, supervise lineage activities, and maintain the lineage genealogies. The first genealogy appeared in 1662, and by the time of the last update in 1921, 28 editions covering a period of two and half centuries had been produced. The recorded population increased from about 1,000 people to 200,000, with 50,000 were alive in 1921. So far, records of 80,000 individuals from the principle imperial line have been included in a computer database, and the research findings reported are mainly derived from these data. See Lee et al (1993).

to the genealogy, two men reached an age of 100 and 3 survived to 102. In addition to that, there are also 13 men who were recorded to have reached an age between 95 and 100. For all these people, detailed dates of birth and death are available, listed in Table 3.

Table 3. Dates of birth and death for those surviving to age 95

Person ID	Generation	Birth date	Death date	Age at death
1	4	31.07.1666	18.06.1766	99.9
2	6	18.02.1710	21.01.1813	102.9
3	6	21.11.1672	13.02.1775	102.2
4	6	10.01.1711	05.09.1807	96.7
5	6	10.03.1693	02.07.1795	102.3
6	6	04.10.1731	06.03.1829	97.4
7	6	14.07.1723	27.04.1819	95.8
8	7	11.12.1696	13.11.1797	100.9
9	7	01.02.1699	12.11.1794	95.8
10	7	11.02.1719	05.11.1815	96.7
11	7	19.01.1732	24.09.1828	96.7
12	7	08.06.1726	13.08.1823	97.2
13	7	30.06.1729	15.07.1829	100.0
14	8	13.09.1724	26.04.1820	95.6
15	8	18.12.1741	11.03.1840	98.2
16	8	02.04.1731	24.04.1828	97.1
17	8	22.01.1733	24.09.1828	95.7
18	9	22.09.1814	11.11.1910	96.1

Source: The Qing Imperial Genealogy. The data are provided by Feng Wang and James Lee.

In the population selected from the Wang Genealogy and the population recorded in the Qing Imperial Genealogy, the proportion of those surviving to very old ages, as has been addressed, is relatively high. Some researchers may accordingly feel uncertain about the longevity records because at very old ages the mortality pattern observed in these selected populations is not as "regular" as that suggested by the model life table. In this respect, two more points need to be added.

Firstly, if the relatively high proportion of those surviving to very high ages is primarily caused by the over-representation of those very old rather than by people exaggerating their ages, the validity of the record longevity will not be affected. Secondly, although model life tables have been widely used and indeed the first section of this chapter is primarily based on the Coale-Demeny model life tables, we should not rely on only the model life tables to judge whether the mortality pattern found in a population is reliable. This is particularly important in the study of mortality patterns at very old ages, since the "regular" mortality patterns mapped by model life tables, especially those under very high mortality, are largely obtained through theoretical modelling rather than empirical investigation (because of the lack of reliable empirical data).

Acknowledgement

This research, which was partly funded by a grant from the Alfred P. Sloan Jr Foundation to the University of Minnesota and by a grant from the U.S. National Institute on Aging to Duke University and Odense University Medical school, has been conducted in the Cambridge Group for the History of Population and Social Structure and the East-West Center of Hawaii. I would like to acknowledge the help and support from the above institutions. I would also like to thank Peter Laslett, James Vaupel, James Lee and Feng Wang for their help and comments.

Literature

Barinaga, M. 1991. How long is the human life-span. *Science*, 254:936-938.

Barinaga, M. 1992. Mortality: overturning received wisdom. *Science*, 258:398-399.

Carey, J.R., P. Liedo, D. Orozco, and J.W. Vaupel. 1992. Slowing of mortality rates at older ages in large Medfly cohorts. *Science*, 258:457-461.

Coale, A., and P. Demeny. 1983. Regional model life tables and stable populations. *Academic Press*, New York.

Gompertz, B. 1825. On the nature of the function expressive of the law of human mortality. In Smith, D., and N. Keyfitz (ed.). 1977. *Mathematical Demography. Springer-Verlag*, Berlin.

Kannisto, V. 1988. On the survival of centenarians and the span of life. *Population Studies*, 42:389-406.

Kannisto, V., J. Lauritsen, A.R. Thatcher, and J.W. Vaupel. 1994. Reduction in mortality at advanced ages. *Population and Development Review 20, No. 4.*

Lee, J. et al. 1993. The last emperors, an introduction to the demography of the Qing (1644-1911) imperial lineage. In Reher, D., and R. Schofield, (ed.). Old and new methods in historical demography. *Clarendon Press*, Oxford.

Lee, J. et al. 1994. Infant and child mortality among the Qing nobility, implications for two types of positive checks. *Population Studies 48:395-411.*

Liu, T-J. 1992. Lineage population and socio-economic changes in the Ming-Ch'ing periods. *The Institute of Economics, Academia Sinica*, Taipei.

Thatcher, A.R. 1992. Trend in numbers and mortality at high ages in England and Wales. *Population Studies*, 46:411-426.

Vaupel, J., and H. Lundström. 1994. The future of mortality at older ages in developed countries. In Lutz, W. (Ed.) The future population of the world. *Earthscan Publications Ltd.*, London.

Wilmoth, J.R., and H. Lundström. 1995. Extreme longevity in five countries: Presentation of trends with special attention to issues of data quality. *European Journal of Population*, forthcoming.

Zhao, Z. 1994. Demographic conditions and multi-generation households in Chinese history, results from genealogical research and microsimulation. *Population Studies, 48:413-425.*

Zhao, Z. 1994. Long term mortality patterns in Chinese history, unpublished manuscript.

The Emergence and Proliferation of Centenarians

by James W. Vaupel & Bernard Jeune

In developed countries the number of people celebrating their 100th birthday multiplied several fold from 1875 to 1950 and doubled each decade since 1950. In Denmark, for instance, an average of only 3 individuals reached age 100 in each year of the 1870s, compared with 213 new centenarians in 1990. Table 1 presents statistics on the number and annual rate of growth in number of persons attaining age 100, for 11 developed countries with highly reliable data. On average, the number of new centenarians increased at an annual rate of about 7% between the 1950s and the 1980s. This pace of increase is exceptionally rapid compared with the more stately progress of most populations.

As with any population, the multiplication of centenarians must be due to some combination of earlier changes in fertility, migration, and mortality (Preston and Coale 1982). In particular, the rate of growth in the number of 100-year-olds can be decomposed into the sum of the rate of increase in births 100 years ago, the rate of decrease in the effects of net emigration, and the rate of improvement in survival from birth to 50, 50 to 80, and 80 to 100. In the next section of this chapter we analyze the relative importance of these factors in explaining the proliferation of centenarians. The results indicate that the proliferation of centenarians is mainly due to improved survival from age 80 to 100.

We then turn to an analysis of the emergence of centenarians. Some simple calculations suggest that over the course of human existence the chance of enduring from birth to age 100 may have increased more than 100,000-fold. This radical change is also largely attributable to reductions in death rates at advanced ages. Taken together, our findings about the emergence and proliferation of centenarians challenge the tenet that mortality among the oldest-old is intractable.

Causes of the Proliferation of Centenarians

Our analysis is based on data from the Odense Archive of Population Data on Aging (Kannisto 1994). Most of the data used were compiled and organized by Väinö

Kannisto and Roger Thatcher. Their data were supplemented with data on Sweden compiled by Hans Lundström, on Norway by Jens Olaf Borgan, and on Denmark by Axel Skytthe and Kirill Andreev. The numbers displayed in Table 1 are for those countries and times for which the quality of the data is excellent; there are serious problems of age misreporting in many countries before 1950 and in some countries, including the United States, more recently (Kannisto 1994, Thoms 1873, Condran *et al* 1991).

Table 1: Number and annual rate of growth in number of persons attaining age 100

Country	Number							Annual rate of growth (%)‡		
	1875*	1915†	1950	1960	1970	1980	1990	1950s to 1960s	1960s to 1970s	1970s to 1980s
Austria	...	...	12	21	41	77	137	8	6	6
Belgium	...	...	21	37	82	136	290	4	5	8
Denmark	3	5	22	25	44	103	213	3	9	8
England & Wales	...	74	183	316	684	1244	1971	7	7	6
Finland	1	1	5	6	14	37	87	4	6	11
France	...	...	171	330	663	1178	2063	8	7	6
Japan	...	...	66	91	221	543	1717	6	10	10
Norway	...	15	23	44	73	85	141	1	5	5
Sweden	4	16	31	46	80	172	329	4	7	7
Switzerland	...	...	9	15	40	99	195	6	8	9
West Germany	...	...	...	94	283	616	1626	...	8	9
Total or average	-	-	543	1025	2225	4290	8769	5.1	7.1	7.7
Weighted average§	-	-	-	-	-	-	-	6.3	7.7	7.7

* average number 1870-9; † average number 1911-20; ‡ logarithm of the ratio of the number of persons attaining age 100 in the second time period to the number in the first time period, divided by ten; § weighted by number of centenarians in 1990; ... required data not available; — statistic not appropriate.

We used the decomposition $n = n_o \, a \, s_{50} \, s_{80} \, s_{100}$, where n is the number of people attaining age 100, n_o is the number of births in the corresponding time period 100 years earlier, a is an adjustment for the effects of migration, s_{50} is the proportion of those born who survive to age 50, s_{80} is the proportion of these survivors who live on to age 80, and s_{100} is the proportion of these octogenarians who endure to celebrate their 100th birthday. Let $ń$ be the rate of growth of n, such that $ń = (dn/dy)/n$, where y denotes time. Defining $ń_o$, $á$, $ś_{50}$, $ś_{80}$, and $ś_{100}$ similarly, it follows (using methods explained in Preston and Coale 1982 and Arthur and Vaupel 1984) that $ń = ń_o + á + ś_{50} + ś_{80} + ś_{100}$. The annual rates of growth in number of births and number attaining age 100 were calculated as the logarithm of the ratio of the number in the second time period to the number in the first time period, divided by the number of years between the time periods.

For Denmark, Norway, and Sweden values of the rate of increase in survival from birth to 50, from 50 to 80, and from 80 to 100 were calculated from cohort lifetable values of annual probabilities of survival, adjusted for migration. For these three countries the adjustment for emigration was calculated as $á = ń - (ń_o + ś_{50} + ś_{80} + ś_{100})$. For the other countries, data were available on the number of people attaining age 80 from 1950 through 1969 and the corresponding number attaining age 100 from 1970 to 1989: the proportion surviving from 80 to 100 was estimated using these data.

In the Scandinavian countries, the cohorts born in the 1880s were larger than those born in the 1870s. Fewer of the members of the later cohorts left their homelands and death rates were lower at all ages. Hence changes in fertility, migration, and mortality at younger and older ages all contributed to the doubling of the number of centenarians between the 1970s and 1980s. The statistics in Table 2 indicate the relative importance of these various changes: the predominant cause of the rise of centenarians is greater survival from age 80 to 100.

We did not have the requisite cohort data for other countries to calculate the effect of all the various factors, but we were able to calculate the contribution of improved survival at advanced ages. In every case, as shown in Table 2, the proliferation of centenarians is mostly due to the reduction in mortality among octogenarians and nonagenarians.

The Emergence of Centenarians

Life expectancy summarizes the harshness of a mortality regime. Over most of the course of human existence life expectancy hovered between 20 and 30 years; even in Western Europe life expectancy did not reach 40 until after 1800 and 50 until after 1900. In many of the countries in Table 1, female life expectancy is now about 80 years; in Japan, female life expectancy is above 82. An analysis of how the chance of surviving to age 100 varies as life expectancy increases from 20 to 80 provides, therefore, a long-term perspective on the emergence of centenarians.

Table 2: Annual average rate of growth from the 1970s to 1980s in the number attaining age 100 and the proportion of this rate of growth due into improved survival from age 80 to 100 and other factors

Country	Average annual rate of growth (in %) from the 1970s to 1980s in the number attaining age 100	Proportion (in %) of this rate of growth due to:				
		Improved survival from:			Decrease in net emigration	Increase in births from the 1870s to 1880s
		age 80 to age 100	age 50 to age 80	birth to age 50		
Austria	5.7	60	...	...	...	...
Belgium	7.8	80	...	...	...	...
Denmark	7.7	66	13	5	0	16
England & Wales	5.8	72	...	...	...	...
Finland	11.2	81	...	...	...	...
France	6.3	73	...	...	...	...
Japan	10.2	67	...	...	...	...
Norway	5.1	65	10	8	3	14
Sweden	7.1	66	12	10	9	4
Switzerland	9.2	73	...	...	...	...
West Germany	9.1	72	...	...	...	...

... data not available.

We based our analysis on data from the female "model West" lifetables estimated by Coale and Demeny, who studied hundreds of lifetables to determine the relationship between the level of life expectancy and the age-trajectory of mortality (Coale and Demeny 1983). Although the Coale-Demeny lifetables are a widely-used demographic standard, our results should be interpreted with caution because few reliable statistics are available concerning levels of mortality among the very old under conditions when life expectancy was low. The lower life expectancy is, the greater the tendency for age exaggeration at older ages (Kannisto 1994, Thoms 1873, Condran et al 1991). This may result in underestimates of death rates at older ages (because many of the alleged older people were actually younger).

Coale and Demeny were aware of data limitations at older ages and relied on a formula to extrapolate death rates from age 80 to age 105. They tested the formula against what they considered to be reliable lifetables, but even these tables are questionable. Their formula is based on the assumption that death rates increase exponentially between ages 80 and 105, attaining an estimated value at age 105. Although this assumption is questionable, so little is known about the age-trajectory of mortality at advanced ages when life expectancy is low that it is not clear whether the Coale-Demeny estimates produce overestimates or underestimates of the probability of surviving to 100. Wilmoth, elsewhere in this monograph, develops a rich array of alternative estimates.

Because of the bias caused by greater age overstatement in populations with shorter life expectancies, the probabilities of survival from age 50 to 80, from 80 to 100, and from birth to 100 in high-mortality regimes may be even lower than the Coale-Demeny data suggest. The seriousness of the problem of age exaggeration can be illustrated by examples from two countries generally considered to have highly reliable vital statistics, Sweden and Norway. Swedish statistics report twice as many Swedes in their 80s and four times in their 90s per million population in 1750 than in 1850 (Sundbärg 1907). In Norway 197 persons are reported as having attained age 100 in the 1870s: this figure is more than 5 times the numbers reported for more populous Denmark and Sweden. The relatively slow rate of growth in the number of centenarians in Norway (Table 1) and the relatively slow rate of improvement in survival from 80 to 100 (Table 2) may be artifacts of decreasing age exaggeration.

Although questionable, results based on the Coale-Demeny estimates are suggestive. Under the most brutish conditions, with a female life expectancy at birth of 20 years (and a remaining life expectancy at age 5 of 37 years), the odds against attaining age 100 are roughly 20 million to 1. When life expectancy at birth increases to 30 years and to 40 years, these odds fall to 700,000 to 1 and 80,000 to 1. Under current mortality rates in the countries with female life expectancies of about 80 years, two women in 100 will survive a century or more. Hence as life expectancy increases four-fold, from 20 to 80, the chance of surviving 100 years swells 400,000-fold. (Zhao, in this monograph, also used the Coale-Demeny estimates to derive the chances of survival to advanced ages: see, in particular, his Figure 1).

This enormous rise in survival chances is largely attributable to an increase in the probability of an octogenarian becoming a centenarian. As life expectancy increases from 20 to 80, the chance of surviving from birth to age 50 grows about 5-fold and the chance of surviving from 50 to 80 increases roughly 15-fold. Remarkable as these changes are, they are dwarfed by the 5,000-fold multiplication of the chance of surviving from 80 to 100.

Let s be the probability of survival from some age to some later age, e.g. from

80 to 100. If the force of mortality (hazard of death) is reduced or increased by the same factor α over all ages in the interval, then the chance of survival becomes s^{α}. Suppose α is 0.5. If s is 0.01, then s^{α} is 0.1, an improvement of 10-fold. If s is 0.000001, then s^{α} is 0.001, an improvement of 1000-fold. Boldsen (in this monograph) suggests that mortality between ages 50 and 100 may have been 8 times higher in Medieval Denmark than in Denmark today. The chance of surviving from 50 to 100 today is roughly 1 in 100, so the chance then would have been roughly 10^{-16}. These calculations illustrate the leverage changes in mortality can have on changes in survival over age intervals with low survival.

Before about 2000 BC, the number of births per year was under 1 million; until roughly 1000 AD annual global births ran at less than 10 million; only since 1970 have more than 100 million babies been added to the human population each year (McEvedy and Jones 1978). If the chance of surviving to age 100 is about 1 in 20 million when life expectancy is 20 and about 1 in 80,000 when life expectancy is 40 (a level not reached in Western Europe until the early 19th century), then centenarians must have been exceedingly rare in most countries before the modern era. Nearly all of the hundreds of Danish centenarians (and super-centenarians) reported in the 18th century are probably tales: in most years before 1800 there may have been no genuine celebration in Denmark of a 100th birthday (Jeune 1994, Skytthe and Jeune and Jeune in this monograph). More generally, unless there is some secret of longevity that has enabled some humans to transcend the death rates that governed the fate of nearly all their contemporaries, most accounts of centenarians in earlier centuries must be inaccurate (Thoms 1873).

Gerontological research - and much health policy - has been guided by the notions that aging is an intrinsic, intractable process, that deaths at advanced ages are "natural", and that little can be done to increase survival among the oldest-old (Fries 1980, Olshansky *et al* 1990). Far from being fixed, however, death rates after age 80 have declined considerably (Kannisto 1994, Kannisto *et al* 1994). The emergence and proliferation of centenarians dramatically illustrates the improvement in the life chances of octogenarians and nonagenarians. Because half of female and a third of male deaths in developed countries now occur after age 80, the plasticity of survival at advanced ages is of considerable significance. If the present pace of improvement in old-age survival persists, then it will be as likely for a child today to reach age 100 as it was for a child born eight decades ago to reach age 80 (Vaupel and Gowan 1986).

Acknowledgement

We thank Väinö Kannisto, Peter Laslett, Hans Lundström, Jim Oeppen, Richard Smith, Richard Suzman, A. Roger Thatcher, Shripad Tuljapurkar, Kenneth Wachter, John Wilmoth, and Anthony Wrigley for suggestions, and Kirill Andreev and Wang Zhenglian for research assistance. Supported by grants from the Danish Research Councils, the U.S. National Institute on Aging (grant AG08761), and the Wellcome Trust.

Literature

Arthur, W.B., and J.W. Vaupel. 1984. Some General Relationships in Population Dynamics. *Population Index* 50:214-226.

Coale, A.J., and P. Demeny. 1983. Regional Model Life Tables and Stable Populations. *Academic Press, New York*.

Condran, G.A., C.L. Himes, and S.H. Preston. 1991. Old-Age Mortality Patterns in Low-Mortality Countries: An Evaluation of Population and Death Data at Advanced Ages, 1950 to the Present. *Population Bull. of the U.N.* 30:23.

Fries, J.F. 1980. Aging, Natural Death, and the Compression of Morbidity. *N.E.J. of Medicine* 303:130.

Jeune, B. 1994. Centenarians - tail or tale? *Gerontologi og Samfund* 10(1),4 [in Danish; English translation available from author].

Kannisto, V. 1994. Development of Oldest-Old Mortality. 1950-1990: Evidence from 28 Developed Countries. *Odense University Press*, Odense, Denmark.

Kannisto, V., J. Lauritsen, A.R. Thatcher, and J.W. Vaupel. 1994. Reductions in Mortality at Advanced Ages: Several Decades of Evidence from 27 Countries. *Population and Development Review* 20:793.

McEvedy, C., and R. Jones. 1978. Atlas of World Population History. *Allen Lane*, London.

Olshansky, S.J, B.A. Carnes, and C. Cassel. 1990. In Search of Methuselah: Estimating the Upper Limits of Human Longevity. *Science* 250:634.

Preston, S.H., and A.J. Coale. 1982. Age Structure, Growth, Attrition, and Accession: a New Synthesis. *Population Index* 48:217-59.

Sundbärg, G. 1907. Bevölkerungsstatistik Schwedens 1750-1900. *Swedish Central Bureau of Statistics*, Stockholm, reprinted 1970.

Thoms, W.J. 1873. Human Longevity, Its Facts and Its Fictions. *John Murray*, London.

Vaupel, J.W., and A.E. Gowan. 1986. Passage to Methuselah: Some Demographic Consequences of Continued Progress against Mortality. *American Journal of Public Health* 76:430.

A Note on Some Historical Data on Old Age Mortality

by A. Roger Thatcher

The main purpose of this brief factual note is to bring together a selection of historical data which seem to the author to provide an interesting long-term perspective on the changes in the force of mortality at high ages since the 17th century.

As a by-product, the data can also be used to produce an estimate of the proportion of people who might have been expected to survive from birth in 1700 to reach age 100 in 1800. It is of interest that this is consistent with the estimates given by Zhao and by Vaupel and Jeune elsewhere in this monograph, and which they derived from model life tables with a life expectancy at birth of between 35 and 40 years.

The historical data

The data which are used in this Note relate to the following periods, starting from the present and working backwards:

(a) England and Wales in 1980-1990. For ages 0-85, the figures are derived from English Life Table No 14. For ages 85 and over they are derived by an extension of the method of extinct generations (Thatcher, 1992).

(b) England and Wales in 1841. The figures are derived from English Life Table No 1, which was compiled by William Farr and published by the Registrar General (1843).

(c) Halley's life table for Breslau in 1687-1691. Halley's life table is reproduced and discussed by Karl Pearson (1978) and by Anders Hald (1990).

(d) British Members of Parliament who died from 1550 onwards. The data on ages at death of British Members of Parliament (M.P.s) are the subject of an on-going study by Peter Razzell, who has published some preliminary results (Razzell, 1993, 1994). Further results are expected from a joint study by Peter

Razzell and Jim Oeppen. The particular figures in Table 1, relating to M.P.s who died at ages 50 and over in the periods 1550-1699, 1700-1799 and 1800-1875, and whose ages at death were known, were calculated by Julia Hynes from data provided by Peter Razzell and the History of Parliament Trust.

The data for M.P.s who entered Parliament before 1660 are not as reliable as the later material, and of course there are problems in estimating life table values from ages at death. Thus the M.P. figures should be regarded as preliminary, pending the forthcoming study by Razzell and Oeppen. They are, however, based on far more data than the comparable estimates for the British aristocracy (Hollingsworth 1977).

Results

Tables 1-3 summarise the relevant survival functions and the derived forces of mortality, averaged over 5-year age groups. These were calculated by the formula

$$5\mu = \ln\left(\frac{l_x}{l_{x+5}}\right)$$

where μ is the average force of mortality between ages x and x+5, and where l_x and l_{x+5} are the numbers surviving to these ages.

Figure 1 illustrates some of the survival curves. Figure 2 shows the changes of mortality over time between the successive groups of M.P.s. Figure 3, in which Halley's life table and the English life tables are plotted down to the age range 30-35, shows the most comprehensive perspective of all.

The probability of survival to age 100

Halley's life table does not start from the exact age 0, but the value of l_0 has been reconstructed by Bockh and is given by Hald (1990) as 1238. Using this, we find from Halley's table that the probabilities of survival at Breslau in 1687-91 were 0.279 from age 0 to age 50, and 0.118 from age 50 to age 80. (The Members of Parliament give 0.080 from age 50 to age 80 in 1550-1699 and 0.135 in 1700-1799). In order to estimate the probability of survival from age 80 to age 100, we take the average value of the force of mortality in this age range as 0.4, which is a reasonable extrapolation of the curves in Figure 3. This implies that the probability of survival from 80 to 100 would be about 1 in 3,000. On combining all these estimates, we find that the probability of survival from age 0 to age 100, for a life table cohort born in 1700, comes to about 1 in 100,000. This is consistent with the estimates derived by Zhao and by Vaupel and Jeune from the model life tables.

Literature

Hald, A. 1990. A history of probability and statistics and their applications before 1750. *Wiley*, New York.

Hollingworth, T.H. 1977. Mortality in the British peerage families since 1600. *Population, special number*.

Pearson, K. 1978. The history of statistics in the 17th and 18th centuries. *Griffin*, London.

Razzell, P. 1993. The growth of population in eighteenth century England: a critical reappraisal. *Journal of Economic History; 53:743-771*.

Razzell, P. 1994. Essays in English Population History. *Caliban Books*, London.

Registrar General. 1843. Fifth report of the Registrar General. *HMSO*, London.

Thatcher, A.R. 1992. Trends in numbers and mortality at high ages in England and Wales. *Population Studies; 46:411-426*.

Table 1: Survivors reaching ages 50 and over

M.P.s 1550-1699			English Life Table No. 1, 1841 Males		
	l_x			l_x	
50	3120	1.000000	50	23376	1.000000
55	2704	0.866667	55	21355	0.913544
60	2150	0.689103	60	18808	0.804586
65	1591	0.509936	65	15589	0.666881
70	1070	0.342949	70	11823	0.505775
75	597	0.191346	75	7867	0.336542
80	249	0.079808	80	4316	0.184634
85	74	0.023718	85	1780	0.076146
90	18	0.005769	90	481	0.020577
95	2	0.000641	95	69	0.002952
100	1	0.000321	100	7	0.000299
105	1	0.000321	104	1	0.000043
M.P.s 1700-1799			English Life Table No. 1, 1841 Females		
	l_x			l_x	
50	3051	1.000000	50	23245	1.000000
55	2686	0.880367	55	21441	0.922392
60	2262	0.741396	60	19188	0.825468
65	1744	0.571616	65	16263	0.699634
70	1257	0.411996	70	12708	0.546698
75	790	0.258931	75	8797	0.378447
80	412	0.135038	80	5082	0.218628
85	162	0.053097	85	2241	0.096408
90	56	0.018355	90	659	0.028350
95	9	0.002950	95	105	0.004517
			100	9	0.000387
			104	1	0.000043
M.P.s 1800-1875			Halley, Breslau 1687-1691		
	l_x			l_x	
50	3085	1.000000	50	346	1.000000
55	2880	0.933549	55	292	0.843931
60	2579	0.835981	60	242	0.699422
65	2213	0.717342	65	192	0.554913
70	1742	0.564668	70	142	0.410405
75	1166	0.377958	75	88	0.254335
80	653	0.211669	80	41	0.118497
85	273	0.088493	84	19	0.054913
90	65	0.021070			
95	9	0.002917			
100	2	0.000648			

Table 2: Mortality of British M.P.s since 1550
Average force of mortality in 5-year age groups

Age group	M.P.s 1550-1699	M.P.s 1700-1799	M.P.s 1800-1875	England & Wales males 1980-1990
50-	0.0286	0.0255	0.0138	0.0079
55-	0.0459	0.0344	0.0221	0.0138
60-	0.0602	0.0520	0.0306	0.0227
65-	0.0793	0.0655	0.0479	0.0365
70-	0.1167	0.0929	0.0803	0.0587
75-	0.1749	0.1302	0.1160	0.0930
80-	0.2427	0.1867	0.1744	0.1432
85-	0.2827	0.2124	0.2870	0.2039
90-	0.4394	0.3656	0.3954	0.2961
95-				0.4156
100-				0.5401

Table 3: Average force of mortality in 5-year age groups

Age group	British M.P.s 1550-1699	Halley's Life Table 1687-1691	English Life Table No.1 males 1841	England & Wales males 1980-1990
30-		0.0161	0.0108	0.0010
35-		0.0193	0.0123	0.0014
40-		0.0228	0.0140	0.0023
45-		0.0275	0.0159	0.0043
50-	0.0286	0.0339	0.0181	0.0079
55-	0.0459	0.0376	0.0254	0.0138
60-	0.0602	0.0463	0.0375	0.0227
65-	0.0793	0.0603	0.0553	0.0365
70-	0.1167	0.0957	0.0815	0.0587
75-	0.1749	0.1528	0.1201	0.0930
80-	0.2427		0.1771	0.1432
85-	0.2827		0.2617	0.2039
90-	0.4394		0.3884	0.2961
95-			0.4576	0.4156
100-				0.5401

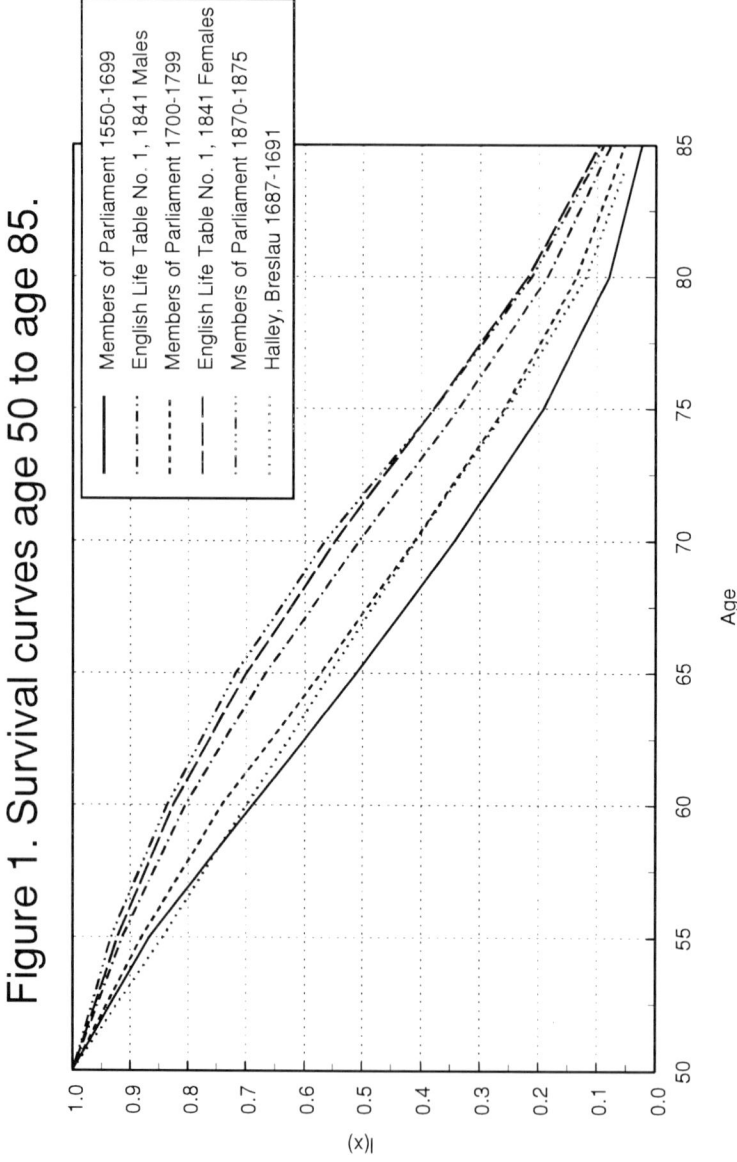

Figure 1. Survival curves age 50 to age 85.

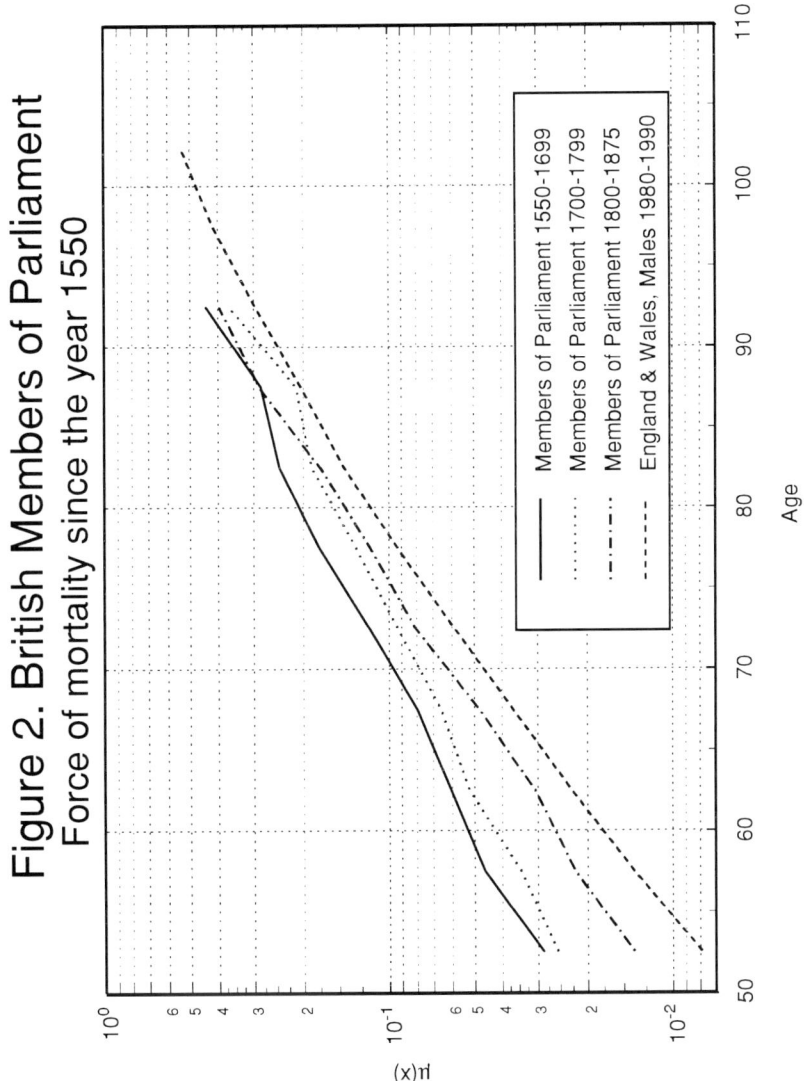

Figure 2. British Members of Parliament
Force of mortality since the year 1550

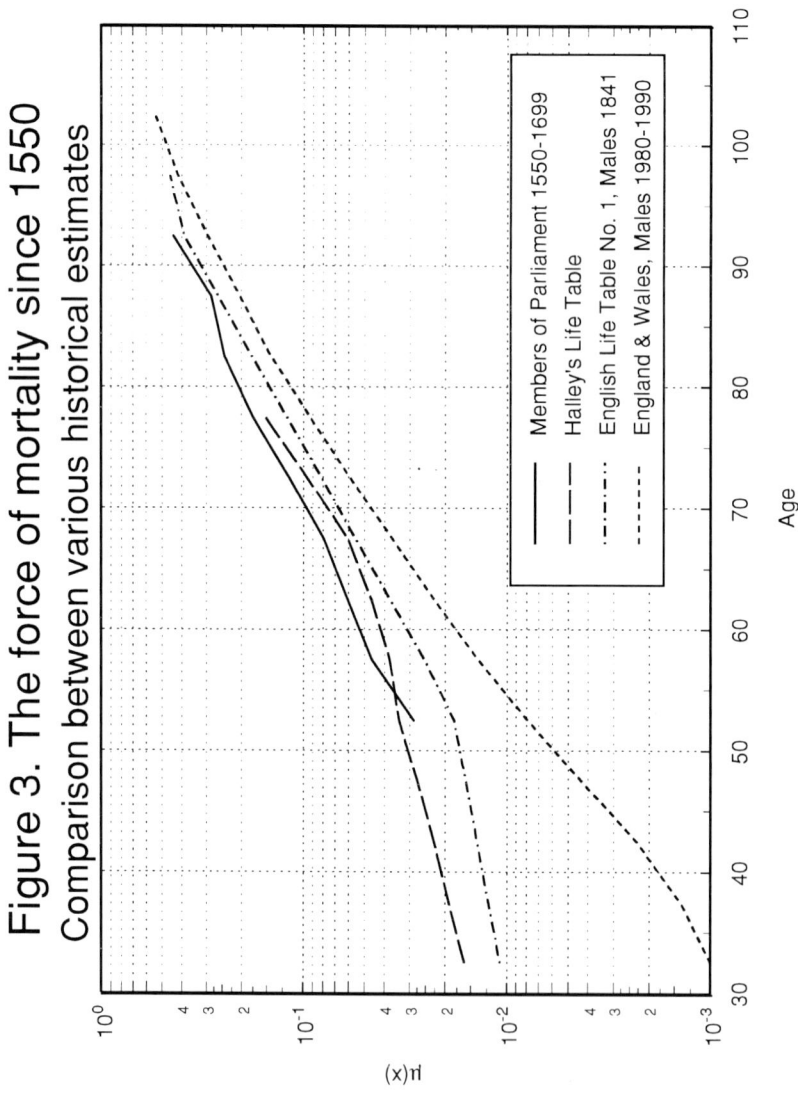

Figure 3. The force of mortality since 1550
Comparison between various historical estimates

The Earliest Centenarians: A Statistical Analysis

by John R. Wilmoth

When did the first centenarians live? It is well documented that the number of centenarians in industrialized countries has increased dramatically during this century (Kannisto 1988, Thatcher 1981, 1992, Vaupel and Jeune, this monograph). Is it conceivable that at some earlier moment in human history there were no individuals who achieved this milestone age? Or, to borrow a phrase from Vaupel and Jeune, when did the "emergence of centenarians" occur? Are centenarians a product of the enormous mortality decline that accompanied industrialization?

Some authors have speculated that centenarians may have been rare or even non-existent prior to the industrial era. For example, based on the observed trend in the maximum reported age at death in Sweden during 1861-1990, Wilmoth and Lundström (1995) speculated that "true centenarians may have been quite rare in the pre-industrial period." Similarly, Jeune (1994 and this monograph) put forth the more daring hypothesis that no humans lived to age 100 before 1800, or to 110 before 1950. Unfortunately, direct tests of these hypotheses are nearly impossible, since accurate records of age at death are usually available only for modern populations. In this chapter we attempt to test these hypotheses using statistical models based on plausible scenarios of adult mortality in the period prior to the mortality decline of the past 250 years.

To accomplish this task, we must address several preliminary questions. First, in the absence of direct evidence, how can the concept of the "emergence of centenarians" be defined and operationalized in a practical yet meaningful fashion? Second, how can we model the age pattern of pre-industrial mortality, especially in the late adult age range (since this is the age range that most affects the probability of survival to age 100)? Third, what are plausible levels and patterns of pre-industrial mortality?

In this chapter, we propose two definitions of the "emergence of centenarians" and demonstrate that our predictions about the timing of that emergence are similar for both definitions. We also suggest that the age pattern of adult mortality can be modeled using the Gompertz-Perks family of curves. We derive evidence about the levels and patterns of pre-industrial mortality from a detailed analysis of model life tables and from a review of existing studies of high-mortality populations.

Combining these various components, we conclude that it is likely that the emergence of centenarians preceded the industrial revolution by several thousand years. There is very little evidence to suggest that the trend in human life expectancy rose (or fell) significantly during the agricultural era. Therefore, the emergence of centenarians during this period must be attributed to the gradual rise in population size, which slowly increased the probability that centenarians, although extremely rare worldwide, should have been observed with some minimal regularity. So defined, our best guess is that the emergence of centenarians occurred once world population rose to about 100 million around 2500 B.C. at the time of the first great civilizations of the ancient world.

The Emergence of Centenarians

Given complete and accurate information about the lifetimes of all individuals who have ever lived, it would be possible to identify a precise date when the first person attained the age of 100 years. Lacking this information, however, we must resort to statistical models that allow us to predict when the earliest centenarians might have lived. These models can not yield precise dates for exact events. Rather, they are used to derive the probability of a given event or an expected number of occurrences within a specified time period.

From a historical perspective, we might say that the emergence of centenarians occurred once the probability that all subsequent birth cohorts should have yielded at least one centenarian was above some level. This definition still requires important choices, however. Do we mean single-year or 100-year birth cohorts, for example? And do we want to require that the event occurs with at least even odds ($p \geq 0.5$) or with virtual certainty ($p \geq 0.99$)? In our calculations, we discovered that the latter choice was not terribly important: most models that offered even odds (or better) of at least one centenarian per cohort predicted, moreover, that a centenarian would be observed with virtual certainty. Thus, we chose the stricter requirement.

The choice of a cohort boundary was more arbitrary. We reasoned that the relevant issue was when centenarians became sufficiently common that they would have been observed at least on occasion worldwide, and it seemed reasonable to equate "on occasion" with "at least once per century". Thus, we propose to examine whether, during a given era, it is likely that there would have been at least "occasional centenarians." Formally, we will state that there were occasional centenarians in some time period if, for a given model of mortality and estimated population size, the probability of observing at least one centenarian per century was 0.99 or more. This definition does not insure that there would always have been one living centenarian on the planet. It does mean, however, that the folklore of a single person who was reputed to have attained this age could not be dismissed as utterly implausible (although it might still be correct to dismiss a multitude of such reports as fallacious). It also means that the phenomenon of being a centenarian was never too far (in a temporal sense) from any living human during this time period.

With this definition, we still face an additional complication due to the fact that multiple mortality scenarios may be considered plausible for a given historical period. Also, although it is substantially less important than the mortality regime, we can estimate the historical size of the world population only within a range. It is possible, therefore, that we could have a number of conflicting indications about whether there were occasional centenarians in some time period. For this reason, in order to assert that centenarians had emerged by some date, we require that there be a "preponderance of evidence" for occasional centenarians from that time onward. Specifically, when considering multiple mortality scenarios, we require that three fourths of them provide a positive indication for occasional centenarians in order to proclaim the emergence of centenarians.

Thus, our first definition of the emergence of centenarians can be summarized as follows: the historical emergence of centenarians is said to have occurred if a preponderance of the available evidence (at least three quarters of the plausible mortality scenarios) indicates with virtual certainty ($p \geq 0.99$) that centenarians must have been observed at least occasionally (no less than once per century).

A second definition of the "emergence of centenarians" relies on the expected number of living centenarians, rather than the probability of survival within a cohort. One reasonable criterion for "emergence" is to require that the expected number of centenarians in the world be at least one. Clearly, this criterion is more strict than requiring at least one centenarian per century. Again, we will consider a range of plausible mortality scenarios, and we will require a "preponderance of evidence" as proof of the "emergence of centenarians."

Using stable population theory, it is possible to compute the expected prevalence of centenarians in the population for a given mortality scenario. Multiplying this number by the estimated population size gives the expected number of living centenarians. Because it is based on a single number (either the prevalence estimate or the expected number of centenarians) rather than a dichotomous indicator variable, this definition is somewhat more amenable to simulation studies than the first definition. A range of plausible mortality scenarios produces a distribution of prevalence estimates. If three quarters of the prevalence estimates predict at least one centenarian in a given time period, then we say, by our second definition, that the emergence of centenarians has occurred.

Gompertz-Perks Family of Mortality Curves

In order to model the probabilities or expectations described in the previous section, we need a model of adult mortality. All mortality curves considered in this chapter fall within the Gompertz-Perks family. This choice can be justified by a combination of theoretical arguments and empirical evidence.

Formulas

The well-known Gompertz mortality curve is given by the simple formula,

$$\mu(x) = ae^{bx} \tag{1}$$

where $a > 0$ and $b > 0$. The Gompertz curve represents the age-dependent component of mortality and is justified, in part, by the statistical theory of extreme values (Gumbel 1937, 1958, Aarssen and de Haan 1994). When plotted in a logarithmic scale, the Gompertz curve rises linearly with age (Figure 1a), thus mimicking one of the most commonly observed features of empirical mortality curves.

In Makeham's formula, a small modification consists of adding a constant parameter to the Gompertz curve:

$$\mu(x) = c + ae^{bx} \tag{2}$$

where $c \geq 0$. The constant, c, represents the level of "background mortality" that is the result of age-independent risks (Gavrilov and Gavrilova 1991, Horiuchi and Wilmoth 1994). Compared to the Gompertz curve, the Makeham curve bends upward at lower ages because it is bounded by a lower asymptote of c (Figure 1b). The importance of the background mortality constant in models of human mortality is well documented. Even Gompertz had speculated about the existence of this second component of adult mortality (Jordan 1975). In recent empirical work, furthermore, it has been demonstrated that a decrease in the age-independent background component has been a major contributing factor to the overall decline of adult mortality during the last century (Gavrilov and Gavrilova 1991).

At the highest ages, it is now well-documented that mortality curves tend to rise less than exponentially (Horiuchi and Coale 1990, Kannisto 1994), suggesting a logistic form, such as contained in Beard's formula:

$$\mu(x) = \frac{ae^{bx}}{1 + vae^{bx}} \qquad (3)$$

where $v \geq 0$. Such a form for the mortality curve is also justified by theoretical arguments, whereby the less-than-exponential increase at advanced ages may reflect either the influence of population heterogeneity and differential selection, or the workings of a multiply redundant system (Yashin *et al.* 1993, Gavrilov and Gavrilova 1991, Horiuchi and Wilmoth 1994). Compared to Gompertz' law, the Beard formula produces a curve that bends over at advanced ages, bounded by an upper asymptote of $1/v$ (Figure 1c).

Combining these two modifications to the Gompertz curve yields Perks' formula:

$$\mu(x) = \frac{c + ae^{bx}}{1 + vae^{bx}} \qquad (4)$$

This formula produces a curve that deviates from the Gompertz at both younger and older adult ages (Figure 1d). The Perks' curve contains an inflection point in late adulthood that should move upward as mortality falls (Horiuchi and Wilmoth 1994). The graphs shown in Figure 1 are drawn using the average values of these four parameters for the simulations of the base model described later in this chapter.

Re-parametrization

The full Perks formula contains 4 parameters, a, b, c, and v. Two of these have fairly direct interpretations: c represents the level of background mortality, $1/v$ gives the upper asymptote of the mortality curve, and both are expressed in terms of the force of mortality, $\mu(x)$, in its original scale. The Gompertz parameters, a and b, on the other hand, are more abstract: b is the rate of exponential increase in mortality across the age range in the Gompertz model, but this interpretation is only approximate in the Makeham, Beard, or Perks models; a is the exact force of mortality at age 0 only in the Gompertz model, but even this fact does not aid in interpretation since the model applies to adult mortality alone.

In choosing the input assumptions for the model, it seemed judicious to reparametrize this model so that all 4 parameters lend themselves to more direct interpretations. Since age 50 was (arbitrarily) chosen as a starting point for our models of late adult mortality, e_{50} (remaining life expectancy at age 50) and $_5m_{50}$ (the death rate between ages 50 and 55) were chosen as alternatives for a and b in the above model. Using numerical methods, it is possible to find the unique parameters, a and b, in the above formulas that reproduce a given e_{50} and $_5m_{50}$ (for fixed levels of c and v).[1] Thus, all model assumptions for this study are expressed in terms of e_{50}, $_5m_{50}$, c and v.

Mortality Levels from the Neolithic to the Industrial Period

Having chosen a family of mortality curves, it is also necessary to examine existing evidence regarding mortality levels and patterns during the pre-industrial period. For example, what were typical values of life expectancy at birth or at age 50? Was the age pattern of mortality similar to what we observe in modern life tables? Is there evidence of a secular trend in mortality levels prior to the enormous decline of the past 200 or 300 years?

It is surely accurate to state that none of these questions can be definitively answered, at least based on evidence now available. Furthermore, it is not the purpose of this study to add to the existing body of evidence about pre-industrial mortality levels. Rather, our purpose in this section is to review the available evidence and to extract from it reasonable conclusions about pre-industrial mortality levels and patterns to serve as the basis for the present inquiry. We will draw our mortality assumptions from a combination of sources. In this section, we examine evidence about mortality levels in populations at historically low levels of life expectancy. In the following section, we analyze data from two collections of model

---

[1] Formally, this conversion ought to include some requirement about choosing "compatible" e_{50} and $_5m_{50}$, so that a and b do not come out to be zero or negative. There probably is no easy analytical description of the boundary conditions for this choice, since formulas for life table functions more complicated than $l(x)$ do not exist for the curves in the Gompertz-Perks family. We have not investigated this issue in detail, but it seems likely to be irrelevant to the present study, which is limited to mortality curves that are in most aspects derived from families of model life tables.

life tables to derive relationships that help to determine the age pattern of mortality.

Regarding mortality levels, Table 1 brings together a number of estimates of life expectancy (both at birth and at age 50) in high-mortality populations from a variety of sources. While we believe that this evidence provides a reasonable justification for the assumptions about pre-industrial life expectancy adopted in this chapter, we also acknowledge that the conclusions of this study may need to be revised at some future date if different and better evidence becomes available.

There have been several notable attempts to trace pre-industrial trends in morbidity and mortality. Reliable written records that could be used to document historical mortality patterns are lacking for almost all large populations prior to the industrial period. Historical demographers, however, have attempted to reconstruct various populations using religious or genealogical records. For example, Hollingsworth (1977) computed life tables for the British peerage beginning with the cohort born in 1550 (see Table 1). More recently, Lee et al. (1993) made mortality estimates for the Qing imperial lineage (1644-1911), and Zhao (1994) calculated life tables for the Wang dynasty during 0-1760 A.D. (Lee and his colleagues present their results in graphical form only, and thus we give them here as a range of values with an indication of the long-term trend.) Although these groups may not be representative, the evidence from these studies of elites provides clues about what the mortality experience of the general population may have been.

Another approach for estimating pre-industrial mortality levels and patterns is based on paleodemographic data (mostly, from studies of skeletal remains). The most extensive work in this area is the book by Acsadi and Nemeskeri (1970), which contains life tables for a variety of populations, from early hunter-gatherers to modern industrial societies. Table 1 in this chapter presents life expectancies for populations from four pre-industrial periods (Stone Age, Copper Age, Roman era, and Middle Ages). From among the various tables presented in Acsadi and Nemeskeri's book, here we consider four that were judged to be among the most reliable (Thatcher 1980). Nevertheless, the mortality levels given here may not be typical of the entire time period in question. For example, the Stone Age population with an estimated life expectancy of 21 years was unearthed at two cemeteries on the Maghreb region in Morocco and Algeria. There it appears that burial practices were stable over a period of two centuries, so it may be reasonable to conclude that the paleodemographic data provide an accurate picture of the mortality of that population. A stable community that survived so long during this time period was likely to be advantaged, however, so Acsadi and Nemeskeri reckon that average Stone Age life expectancies were probably lower than 21 years (a conclusion that may or may not be correct).

There are several reasons to be cautious about interpreting literally life tables constructed from paleodemographic data (Sattenspiel and Harpending 1983, Johannson and Horowitz 1986, Paine 1989, Wood *et al.* 1992). Probably the two most important for our purposes are the problems of selection bias and non-stationarity. As suggested above, populations for which reliable paleodemographic data are available may tend to be an advantaged or otherwise unrepresentative sample. Non-stationarity results in biased estimates of life expectancy insofar as the real distribution of deaths in the population does not mirror the hypothetical distribution of deaths in the life table. A population with a stable positive growth rate, for example, would have an average age at death that is lower than the life expectancy of the average individual.

Although these biases may be severe, it is also possible that they may tend to cancel each another. If availability of apparently reliable paleodemographic data is a marker of an advantaged society, then that advantage may be reflected in both lower mortality and a positive growth rate. While the former would contribute to an overestimate of average life expectancies, the latter would lead to an underestimate. It is difficult to speculate without further investigation about whether these two biases might be of similar magnitude. This argument does suggest, however, that paleodemographic studies, in spite of their obvious flaws, may still provide a useful indication of pre-industrial life expectancies.

In speculating about pre-industrial mortality levels, it is also useful to make comparisons to high-mortality populations from more recent times. For this purpose, Table 1 presents data from Indian life tables during the late 19th and early 20th centuries (Davis 1951), as well as estimates for three 19th-century slave populations (John 1988, Roberts 1952, Koplan 1983). The table also gives mortality estimates for a unique group of freed American slaves who returned to Africa to build colonial settlements in Liberia (McDaniel 1992). Life expectancy at birth for these Liberian immigrants is the lowest ever recorded for a human population, due apparently to the enormous toll of tropical diseases for which the immigrants lacked immunity. When life expectancies are calculated conditional on surviving a full year after immigration, however, the Liberian levels are much closer to those observed in other high-mortality populations (at least for life expectancy at birth, e_0). Finally, Table 1 also gives life expectancies for Sweden during 1751-1760, around the beginning of the industrial era, from Breslau during 1687-1691 (Halley's life table), and from England and Wales and the city of Liverpool during 1841 (except the Swedish data, these figures come from Thatcher 1980).

It is difficult to find clear evidence in Table 1 of long-term changes in mortality levels prior to 1600 A.D. Mortality declines during recent centuries are evident in the data for the British peers, the Qing imperial line, and India. For the British peers, this decrease is apparently concentrated in the adult ages, while for the Qing, infancy and childhood appear to have been main loci of change. Over a much longer and earlier time period, however, data for the Wang clan show no evidence of a secular mortality decline. Unfortunately, the genealogical data used in the latter study contain incomplete records of infant and childhood deaths, so reliable estimates of life expectancy at birth are not available. Still, it is worth noting that the absence of a long-term trend in Wang mortality during 0-1760 A.D. is indicated for all ages above 20 years (Zhao 1994).

Thus, although the mortality decline of the past few centuries has been dramatic, there appears to be no solid evidence of significant long-term changes in human life expectancy prior to the 17th century. Cohen (1989) argues eloquently that human health and mortality deteriorated following the transition to agriculture that began around 8000 B.C., although other scholars offer a more cautious interpretation of the existing evidence (Wood *et al.* 1992). During the succeeding 10 millenia, there appear to be no compelling arguments regarding the long-term trend in human mortality prior to around 1600. It is certain that mortality levels fluctuated widely during this period (Flinn 1981), but the evidence, flawed though it may be, provides little suggestion of a long-term trend either upward or downward.

If we accept the theory that mortality trends were essentially flat during most of the agricultural era, we are still faced with the problem of determining the prevailing average level of life expectancy. Based on Table 1, we have adopted a working assumption that the worldwide e_{50} during the agricultural era averaged around 14 years. It seems conceivable that this estimate could be off by a few years in either direction, or that there could have been periodic swings in mortality levels lasting a century or more. Therefore, our analyses in succeeding sections of this chapter always consider a range of plausible life expectancies. Given the available evidence, however, it seems unlikely that e_{50} on a world scale would have dipped below 9 years or risen above 19 years for extended periods during this era.

The justification for assuming that e_{50} had an average value around 14 years in the agricultural era is imperfect but, on balance, a seemingly reasonable conclusion. A simplistic argument is that e_{50} must have averaged around 14 years since that value lies at the midpoint of the range of available estimates (roughly, from 9 to 19 years).

Nevertheless, some of the evidence in Table 1 might suggest that typical values of e_{50} were lower than 14 years. For example, among the results from Acsadi and Nemeskeri, only the Roman life table has an e_{50} above 12 years, but the residents of the Roman empire may have enjoyed an unusually advantageous health environment compared with surrounding peoples and time periods. Thus, the lower values of e_{50} found in the tables for the Copper Age and the Middle Ages could represent more typical levels of pre-industrial life expectancy.

It is quite questionable whether all of the estimates of e_{50} in Table 1 should be read literally, however. In particular, the estimates based on skeletal remains are suspect, since apparently the techniques of age imputation on which they rely produced no evidence of very old individuals. Thus, the life tables for the Stone Age, the Copper Age, and the Middle Ages referred to in Table 1 indicate a zero probability of surviving past ages 78, 76, and 85, respectively. It is worth mentioning that, among the four sets of life expectancies in Table 1 taken from Acsadi and Nemeskeri (1970), only the Roman set was not based on skeletal remains. Rather, this Roman era life table was constructed from tombstone epitaphs and contains a maximum age at death of 100 years. It is less surprising, then, that it alone among these four contains a higher estimate of e_{50}.

We might also argue that the results in Table 1 are biased because elite populations are over-represented. For example, some of the highest estimates of adult life expectancies during the agricultural era are found in the life tables for the Wang dynasty, but these pertain to an elite population whose mortality experience may have been atypical compared to the overall population.[2] On the other hand, the earliest mortality estimates for the British peerage, another elite group, contain an e_{50} of only about 12 years. Therefore, the mortality experience of elites is not necessarily more favorable than the average.

A further piece of evidence that e_{50} should have averaged around 14 years during the agricultural era comes from combining direct mortality estimates with information from model life tables. For example, Table 2 shows the values of e_0 and e_{50} contained in Coale-Demeny model life tables at low levels (Coale and Demeny 1983), and in an alternative set of model life tables constructed by Preston et al. (1993). If we believe that agricultural e_0 was centered in the low to mid twenties (and almost all the available evidence is consistent with this conclusion), then the Coale-Demeny model life tables indicate that e_{50} should have been around 14 years or slightly higher.

At these low levels of life expectancy, however, the Coale-Demeny model life tables are the result an extrapolation from life tables at much higher levels of life expectancy. Indeed, the lowest levels of e_0 in the tables used to construct this set of model life tables were 33.4 years for males and 35.5 years for females (Preston et al. 1993). Thus, the relationships between e_0 and e_{50} in very high mortality populations may be poorly represented by these tables. Some authors have argued, in particular,

---

[2] Although note that, since the estimates of e_{50} for the Wang are around 16-18 years, this would be an advantaged mortality experience even if average values were as high as 14 years.

that the Coale-Demeny tables may overestimate infant mortality at low levels of life expectancy and simultaneously underestimate adult mortality (Bhat 1987, Preston *et al.* 1993). Thus, the values of e_{50} for the Coale-Demeny tables in Table 2 may be too high relative to e_0.

A new set of model life tables, however, seeks to correct this imperfection. Preston *et al.* (1993) computed model life tables at low levels of life expectancy based on interpolation between the raw Liberian life table described earlier (with extremely low life expectancies, as seen in Table 1) and the United Nations General mortality pattern with $e_0 = 35$. The relationship between e_0 and e_{50} for these tables is also shown in Table 2. From these results, if e_0 was around 24 years, then e_{50} should have been around 14 years. Furthermore, in order to obtain an e_{50} as low as 12 years, these model life tables suggest that the average male-female e_0 would need to be around 15 years, a value that seems unrealistically low based on all available historical evidence. In conclusion, then, the evidence from model life tables seems to provide additional support for our assumption that agricultural levels of e_{50} should have been around 14 years on average.

As stated earlier, however, the purpose of this investigation is not to resolve the issue of mortality levels and trends during the agricultural era. Rather, our strategy here is to use existing evidence to derive plausible input assumptions for our models of centenarian prevalence. If these assumptions prove to be incorrect upon consideration of further evidence, the results presented here could simply be modified using the same model with new inputs. Furthermore, since we employ a range of assumptions in this chapter, the reader has the opportunity to arrive at different conclusions without making additional calculations.

Mortality Patterns at Low Life Expectancies from Model Life Tables

Aside from the question of mortality levels, it is also necessary to make assumptions about the relationships that determine the age pattern of mortality. In the Gompertz-Perks model, the mortality curve is fully specified only when a chosen value of e_{50} is accompanied by assumptions regarding $_5m_{50}$, c, and v. Three of these parameters, e_{50}, $_5m_{50}$, and c, tend to be strongly correlated, so they must be chosen in a manner to insure that the resulting mortality curve is plausible. That is, in most known life tables, a given level of e_{50} tends to be associated with a fairly narrow range of values for $_5m_{50}$ and c. If these correlations are ignored in choosing the input parameters, the curve that results may be quite different in character from anything we have thus far observed in populations for which reliable data are available.

Of course, it is possible that mortality curves for pre-industrial populations differed in fundamental ways from the more recent life tables that form the basis of our experience in these matters. In this study, however, we assume that early life tables share the same kinds of empirical relationships between the parameters of the Gompertz-Perks family that are observed in modern life tables. These relationships can best be derived through an analysis of model life tables and are expressed here by a series of regressions. These regression are used to guide the choice of model parameters in the analyses of the following sections.

The two most commonly used sets of model life tables are the Coale-Demeny and U.N. collections (Coale and Demeny 1983, United Nations 1982). Both were developed based on observed empirical relationships among life tables constructed from what were thought to be reliable data. Both collections of model life tables contain a handful of "regions" or "patterns," which represent different typical age schedules of mortality. The Coale-Demeny system contains four regions: North, South, East, and West. The U.N. system contains five patterns: Chilean, Latin American, Far Eastern, South Asian, and General.

As noted earlier, however, few of the life tables used in constructing these two sets of model life tables displayed overall levels of mortality that would be considered very low by historical standards. Among the input tables for the U.N. set, the lowest life expectancies at birth were 37.6 (males) and 40.1 (females). Coale and Demeny had only a few reliable observations of mortality at lower levels of life expectancy: the lowest levels of e_0 in their input tables were 33.4 years for males and 35.5 years for females (Preston *et al.* 1993). In contrast, it is generally assumed that life expectancy in the pre-industrial era was centered in the low to mid twenties (see previous section). Thus, the model life tables used for guiding our choice of model parameters are already based, in part, on extrapolations of the age pattern of mortality outside the range of reliable life tables.[3]

Our first task is to choose values of $_5m_{50}$ and c for a given level of e_{50}. Figure 2 demonstrates the inverse log-linear relationship that is typical for e_{50} and $_5m_{50}$. This graph also shows the linear regression of the model life table values of $\log(_5m_{50})$ on

---

[3]Detailed data for the new model life tables by Preston *et al* (1993) became available to us after the computational analyses of this paper were complete. Due to time constraints, it was not possible to re-compute the regression equations and subsequent simulations including these new tables, which have the advantage of being derived from an interpolation within the range, rather than an extrapolation outside the range, of actual data. It seems unlikely, however, that their inclusion would have changed our results substantially.

e_{50}. The analysis is restricted to model life tables with e_0 below 40 years for the U.N. tables, or levels 1-9 for the Coale-Demeny tables. The data points for females are indicated by upper-case letters; for males, by lower-case letters. This regression explains 84 percent of the original variance in $\log(_5m_{50})$. Three lines are shown in Figure 2: the OLS regression line, and this regression line plus and minus the maximum residual from the regression. In the analyses that follow, the choice of $_5m_{50}$ for a given e_{50} is centered around the value given by this OLS regression line. Alternate values are expressed as the regression estimate plus or minus some proportion of the maximum residual.[4]

The method for choosing values of the background mortality parameter, c, is somewhat more complicated, because it involves a multiple regression. Figure 3 shows simple scatter plots of c against both e_{50} and $_5m_{50}$.[5] Neither of these pairs are as strongly correlated as e_{50} and $\log(_5m_{50})$ (the correlation coefficients are -0.72 for e_{50} and c and 0.85 for $\log(_5m_{50})$ and c, compared to 0.94 for e_{50} and $\log(_5m_{50})$). The best prediction is achieved by regressing c on both e_{50} and $_5m_{50}$, although such a model still only explains 77 percent of the original variance. In some of the analyses that follow, the value for c is assumed to equal either this regression estimate, or the estimate plus or minus some proportion of the maximum residual from the regression.

The fourth parameter of the Gompertz-Perks mortality model, v, determines the upper asymptote of the mortality curve. Unlike the other parameters, however, the values of v that were found by fitting the Perks formula to model life tables did not demonstrate significant or meaningful correlations with the other parameters. In any case, these estimated values of v should not be viewed as reliable, since they are based on model life tables with limited detail regarding the age pattern of mortality in the age range where the effects of this parameter are most evident, in particular, above age 90 or 100. For this reason, in the following analyses, the parameter v was chosen in a more arbitrary fashion, based nevertheless on empirical evidence about typical values of this parameter derived from modern, low-mortality populations.

A fifth mortality parameter is needed when we calculate estimates of centenarian prevalence. Because the Gompertz-Perks model is valid only in the adult age range (in our usage, above age 50), we also need an estimate of survivorship at

---

[4] An alternative method would have been to choose a range of values for $\log(_5m_{50})$ based on multiples of the root mean-squared-error of the regression. If the observations were independent, there would be an elegant statistical theory to support such a choice. In this situation, however, the observations are clearly dependent, so there is no strong rationale for using this technique.

[5] Values of c were estimated by fitting the Perks formula to model life table $_5m_x$ values (above age 50 only) using the method of maximum likelihood.

younger ages. Using standard notation, let $l(50)$ be the proportion surviving from birth to age 50. As before, to obtain a "best estimate" of $l(50)$ (conditional on e_{50}, $_5m_{50}$, and c) we will rely on a regression equation derived from model life tables at low life expectancies. In simulations, the chosen value of $l(50)$ will equal this estimate plus or minus some multiple of the maximum residual from the regression analysis. One complication, however, is that we dropped the life tables for the U.N. Far Eastern pattern before fitting the regression model, since the relationship between $l(50)$ and the other parameters is quite atypical in this case: the values of $l(50)$ for the Far Eastern tables are unusually high, so including them in the model shifts the regression estimate upward and produces rather large residuals. It was thus convenient to eliminate the Far Eastern tables from the main analysis and later to test the importance of this simplification in a sensitivity analysis.

Evidence for an "Occasional Centenarian" prior to 1700

The first question that we will address in this chapter can be stated as follows: Is it plausible that there were individuals who attained the age of 100 years, at least on occasion, during the long period of human history from the Agricultural to the Industrial Revolutions? As a shorthand for this question, we are looking for evidence of an "occasional centenarian" during this period. There is very little reliable historical documentation from this period that might definitively resolve this issue. Thus, our investigation will be based on statistical models, which are used to assess the plausibility that at least a few individuals, on a worldwide basis, might have attained the milestone age of 100 years prior to around 1700.

There are various means of defining, formally, what is meant by the phrase "an occasional centenarian." Statistical models of the kind described in the previous section all yield non-zero estimates of the probability of survival to age 100, and thus they produce non-zero estimates of the expected number of centenarians (however defined) as well. We must choose a threshold level for the probability of observing at least one centenarian during some period. As discussed previously, it seems reasonable to assert that an "occasional centenarian" would mean that at least one person had attained this age (worldwide) during a given century.

Accepting the arbitrary nature of these choices, we thus propose the following formalization of the notion of an occasional centenarian. Let X be a random variable representing the number of individuals who attain age 100 during a given century. Then, for a given mortality scenario, we will say that there is an occasional centenarian during that century if $P[X \geq 1] > 0.99$. In a Poisson probability model, this requirement implies that the expected number of centenarians during this period is at least 4.6. In other words, an average of 5 or more centenarians every 100 years is almost certain to yield at least one centenarian per century.

Figures 4 through 6 summarize the results of this analysis. A brief outline of the steps taken to produce a single data point in Figures 4 through 6 is given below, followed by a more detailed description of each step:

1. Choose a set of four input parameters (e_{50}, $_5m_{50}$, c and v), limiting the choice of input parameters to values that may be considered at least weakly plausible based on mortality patterns in model life tables and other sources.
2. Convert e_{50} and $_5m_{50}$ to a and b (holding c and v constant).
3. Using the Gompertz-Perks model, compute the probability of survival from age 50 to 100, thus $l(100) / l(50)$.
4. Choose an assumption for the initial population size, called N_{50}, which equals the estimated number of persons who attain age 50 (worldwide) during a given century.
5. Following the binomial model, compute the expected number of survivors to age 100, called λ, out of the initial cohort of N_{50}. Thus, $\lambda = N_{50} \frac{l(100)}{l(50)}$.
6. Following the Poisson model, compute the probability of at least one surviving centenarian out of an initial cohort of N_{50} individuals, thus $1 - e^{-\lambda}$. If this probability exceeds 0.99, then a dot corresponding to the assumed parameter values is plotted in Figures 4 through 6 in the appropriate location.

Step 1

The decision to limit assumed values of e_{50} to the range of 9-19 years was based on the evidence presented earlier, which shows that this range includes almost all plausible estimates of mortality levels above age 50 in agricultural populations prior to the mortality decline of the industrial period. We use model life tables to guide our choice of $_5m_{50}$ and c for a given level of e_{50}. For each value of e_{50}, seven levels of $_5m_{50}$ were considered: the regression estimate (see previous section) plus or minus 0.5, 1, or 1.5 times the maximum residual from the regression.

The choices of c used in constructing Figures 4-6 are based partly on the regression model of the previous section and partly on a simpler strategy for obtaining an assumed value of the background mortality parameter. Regression values plus or minus some multiple of the maximum residual sometimes yielded implausible, or even impossible (i.e., negative), values of c. For this reason, one set of calculations in Figures 4-6 is based on the exact regression estimates of c. The other three sets of calculations assume that c is some fixed proportion of the mortality rate between ages 50 and 55, $_5m_{50}$. For the model life tables considered here, this proportion varies from a minimum of 9 percent to a maximum of 63 percent. Thus, calculations based on assumed proportions of 5 and 65 percent represent the extremes of plausibility, while 35 percent is an intermediate value. By choosing the values of c in this fashion, we are also better able to consider the impact of this background mortality parameter on calculated survival probabilities.

The last parameter to be chosen, v, determines the upper asymptote of the mortality curve. As noted before, this asymptote equals $1/v$. Setting $v = 0$ implies that mortality increases in an exponential fashion (hence, with no upper limit) at the highest ages. Setting $v = 1$ implies that the upper asymptote of the $\mu(x)$ curve equals one. The values of v used here can safely be thought to cover the range of plausible levels of this parameter. An upper asymptote of one is a fairly reasonable assumption based on available empirical evidence, although it is important to bear in mind that such evidence that exists is derived from modern, low-mortality populations. The assumptions, $v = 0.5$ and $v = 1.5$, are probably already sufficiently extreme that they cover the plausible range of human experience. The assumption, $v = 0$, is included mostly for comparison purposes and seems much less likely based on evidence from modern life tables.

Step 2

Numerical methods were used to convert e_{50} and $_5m_{50}$ into a and b (for given values of c and v). In brief, the value of b is found by a numerical search algorithm to match the assumed value of e_{50}. On each iteration, the value of a given b is obtained using equation (4) and assuming that $\mu(52.5) = {_5m_{50}}$.

Step 3

The probability of survival from age 50 to 100, thus $l(100) / l(50)$, is calculated using the following formula:

$$\frac{l(x)}{l(y)} = \begin{cases} \left(\dfrac{1 + vae^{bx}}{1 + vae^{by}}\right)^{\frac{1}{b}(c - \frac{1}{v})} e^{-c(x-y)} & \text{if } v > 0 \\ e^{\{-c(x-y) - \frac{a}{b}(e^{bx} - e^{by})\}} & \text{if } v = 0 \end{cases} \qquad (5)$$

Step 4

Assumed population sizes are based on those given in Durand (1977) and shown in Table 3. It is necessary to convert estimates of total population size into N_{50}, which equals the estimated number of persons who attained age 50 during a given century. Three periods were selected for this analysis: circa 8000 B.C., corresponding (roughly) to the beginning of the agricultural era; circa A.D. 0-14, during the Roman Empire; and the 17th century, just prior to the Industrial Revolution.

It is clear from a comparison of Figures 4, 5, and 6 that these calculations are not terribly sensitive to differences in population size: even the very large differences in base population between these three time periods yield rather small differences in the probability of observing an occasional centenarian (in case it is not obvious to the reader, the differences between these three figures are due entirely to differences in assumed population size). Similarly, all plausible population estimates for a single time period produce nearly identical results, so we can comfortably choose a single set of estimates and not worry about the sensitivity of the results to this one parameter choice.

To obtain an assumed value of N_{50} for each time period, we began by observing that the proportion of a population that is age 50 lies within a fairly narrow range under a variety of plausible assumptions about mortality levels and growth rates. For example, considering all model life tables in the Coale-Demeny system with e_0 between 20 and 30 years, and allowing the growth rate in a stable population to fluctuate between -0.5 and +1 percent, the number of individuals who are aged 50 as a proportion of the total population lies in a range of 0.64 to 1.2 percent (the details of these calculations, based on Coale and Demeny 1983, are available from the author upon request). For a single estimate, therefore, it seems reasonable to assume that the number of individuals attaining age 50 *in a single year* equals 0.9 percent of the average total population for that year. For this analysis, however, we have defined N_{50} to be the number of persons who attain age 50 over the period of a century. Thus, multiplying by 100, we will assume that N_{50} equals 0.9 multiplied by the average total population during the century.

For the three time periods in question (circa 8000 B.C., circa A.D. 0-14, and the 17th century), we assume that the average total population size was 8, 300, and 700 million persons (see Table 3). Thus, N_{50} for these three periods was taken to equal 7.2, 270, and 630 million persons. Although these estimates must be considered very rough approximations, they are adequate given the minimal sensitivity of the results to this particular assumption.

Step 5

Calculation of the estimated number of centenarians out of an initial cohort of N_{50} persons is straightforward using the binomial probability model. In this instance, the probability of survival is $l(100) / l(50)$, and thus the expected number of centenarians, λ, equals $N_{50} \frac{l(100)}{l(50)}$.

Step 6

The Poisson model provides a convenient and accurate approximation to the binomial in situations where the population size is large and the probability of "success" is small. Given λ, the expected number of centenarians, the probability of observing at least one centenarian equals $1 - e^{-\lambda}$. If this probability exceeds 0.99, then a dot corresponding to the assumed parameter values is plotted in Figures 4 through 6 in the appropriate location. These figures are drawn in a way that allows us to observe the importance of all four parameters of the Gompertz-Perks mortality model. Each figure contains four graphs, which differ among themselves in the manner of choosing the background mortality parameter, c. In addition, for each combination of e_{50} and $_5m_{50}$ in these graphs, there may be up to four points representing four assumed values of the parameter v (these four points are centered around the assumed value of e_{50}, which in all cases equals a whole number value between 9 and 19 years).

Interpretation

The purpose of Figures 4-6 is to provide information about the mortality conditions that would have been necessary in a given era to yield an occasional centenarian, without yet speculating in a precise manner about what those mortality conditions were. At this point, we are asserting only that overall mortality levels above age 50 in these periods were probably in a range to produce an e_{50} between 9 and 19 years, with associated levels of $_5m_{50}$, c, and v as depicted in these graphs. These three figures make it clear, therefore, that our ultimate conclusions about the existence of occasional centenarians in the pre-industrial era will depend on our assumptions about the actual levels of mortality within this broad range.

These figures provide an illustration of the role of the various model parameters in determining the likelihood of survival to age 100. All four parameters can have important effects on the conclusions emerging from this sort of analysis, although it may be less obvious why each parameter affects survival probabilities in a given manner. Clearly, increasing values of e_{50} are associated with increasing probabilities of survival and thus an increasing likelihood of observing an occasional centenarian. For a given level of e_{50}, however, Figures 4-6 indicate that survival to age 100 is more likely for relatively higher values of $_5m_{50}$. This result can be explained as follows: for a fixed value of e_{50}, a higher value of $_5m_{50}$ is associated with a slower pace of mortality increase with age, thus yielding a higher probability of survival to very advanced ages.

Similarly, it is also evident that higher values of the background mortality parameter, c, (expressed as a percentage of $_5m_{50}$) are associated with a lower probability of survival to age 100. The explanation is somewhat complicated: a higher level of background mortality around age 50 implies a lower level of senescent mortality; above age 50 in this situation, senescent mortality must increase more rapidly in order to match the fixed level of e_{50}, thus yielding a more pronounced die-off at older ages and thus a lower probability of survival to advanced ages. Thus, as seen in Figures 4-6, the likelihood of observing an occasional centenarian diminishes considerably as c increases from 5 to 65 percent of $_5m_{50}$. Typically, the value of c as a percent of $_5m_{50}$ declines as mortality levels drop and life expectancy increases. Thus, the fourth graph in each figure, where c is derived from an OLS regression of c on e_{50} and $_5m_{50}$, is more similar to the graph marked "c = 65%" at low levels of e_{50} and to the graph marked "c = 5%" at high levels of e_{50}.

The importance of the fourth parameter, v, is also evident in Figures 4-6. Since $1/v$ equals the upper asymptote of the age curve of mortality, higher values of v are associated with lower mortality rates at high ages and thus higher probabilities of survival to advanced ages. For this reason, the dots in Figures 4-6 are most often present in the fourth column of each cluster (corresponding to $v = 1.5$) and most often absent in the first column ($v = 0$).

In all three time periods examined in Figures 4-6, it is evident that life expectancies (e_{50}) at the low end of the range considered here imply mortality conditions that could have been too harsh to guarantee at least one centenarian per century. At the other extreme, a relatively high value of e_{50} within this range suggests mortality conditions that would have yielded at least one centenarian per century in almost every conceivable scenario. In between these two extremes, it is difficult to reach any firm conclusions about whether or not there may have been occasional centenarians during these time periods. To develop this discussion further, however, we first need some standard about how to evaluate the information in these figures.

Note that it is possible to have a maximum of 28 dots in these figures for each combination of e_{50} with a given method of deriving c, the background mortality parameter. If all 28 dots are present, we may conclude that an occasional centenarian was extremely likely (i.e., with a probability greater than 0.99) under every plausible mortality scenario at that level of mortality and for that choice of c. If we narrow our focus to the overall mortality level, e_{50}, then there are a total of 4 x 28 = 112 possible dots. Note in Figure 6, for example, that only 5 of these 112 possible dots are missing when e_{50} equals 19. At the other extreme, there are only 50 dots present (thus, less than half) in these graphs when e_{50} equals 9. If we consider that all of these scenarios are equally likely (surely not the case, but a useful simplification for our current purposes), we have a quantitative means of asserting that assumed levels of e_{50} around 19 suggest that there would almost certainly have been at least one centenarian during the 17th century, while levels around 9 indicate that the existence of a single centenarian in this period would have been a possibility although by no means a certainty.

In the middle range of e_{50}, any conclusion about the likelihood of an occasional centenarian depends critically on the assumed values of the other parameters of the mortality model and on population size as well. When e_{50} equals 14, for example, the three figures contain a total of 63, 89, or 90 dots out of the 112 possible (corresponding to the periods around 8000 B.C., A.D. 0-14, and the 17th century, respectively). Thus, for the latter two periods, mortality levels in the middle range would yield an occasional centenarian in more than three fourths of the plausible mortality scenarios. For the earliest time period, however, only about half of the plausible scenarios at this level of e_{50} would produce an occasional centenarian. Therefore, we might reasonably conclude that an e_{50} around 14 years would provide a fairly strong indication (though no guarantee) of occasional centenarians from at least Roman times to the present. In earlier time periods with much smaller population sizes, such as those probably observed at the dawn of the agricultural era, it seems almost equally likely from our vantage point that an e_{50} around 14 years might have yielded at least one centenarian per century, or that centenarians could have been rarer or even non-existent.

In a previous section, we have argued that a life expectancy, e_{50}, around 14 years is a reasonable "best guess" based on available evidence of mortality levels prior to the industrial era. If this estimate is accurate, we might wish to identify more precisely the first time period in which there is a strong indication that there would have been at least an occasional living centenarian. Based on the preceding analysis, we may attempt to identify a population size and corresponding time period where three fourths of the mortality scenarios associated with an e_{50} of 14 years indicate the presence of an occasional centenarian with very high probability. By trial and error, it was determined that a world population of just under 100 million persons would be sufficient to produce such a result. Using Durand's population estimates (see Table 3) and assuming a fairly stable growth rate between 8000 B.C. and A.D. 0-14, such a population size would have been attained sometime during 3000-2000 B.C., thus around the time of the nascent civilizations of the ancient world (for example, the Old Kingdom in Egypt, or the Sumerian era in Mesopotamia).[6]

Arguably, then, centenarians may have been a product, not of industrialization during the past 200 years, but of civilization during the past 5000 years. It was not the trappings of civilization *per se*, however, that would have yielded an increase in the likelihood of observing an occasional centenarian, since there is no evidence that the rise of early civilizations resulted in a reduction in levels of morbidity or mortality, or a corresponding increase in life expectancy (Cohen 1989). Rather, it was the slow growth of world population during this period that accounts for the increasing probability that at least one individual would have attained this milestone age during the course of a single century. It must therefore be considered coincidental that the critical population mass necessary to yield an occasional centenarian at the assumed mortality level (e_{50} around 14 years) was attained around the time of the birth of civilization.

Estimates of Centenarian Prevalence prior to 1700

Our earlier analysis has shown that, under plausible mortality assumptions, at least an occasional individual must have survived to the age of 100 years since the beginnings

---

[6]It is worth noting that the estimates of historical population size by Biraben (1979) suggest that a world population of 100 million may have first been achieved somewhat later, around 1200 B.C. The paucity of reliable data about world population size in this period requires that we acknowledge the uncertainty of our estimated date for the emergence of centenarians, although it does not seem obligatory that we revise our best estimate based on the difference between Biraben's and Durand's figures.

of civilization some 4000-5000 years ago. Another approach to this problem is to estimate the prevalence of centenarians in a stable population under a range of assumptions. Using this approach, we specify an *a prior* distribution for each parameter of the mortality model, and then calculate prevalence estimates by drawing randomly from those distributions. The result is a distribution of estimates of centenarian prevalence. The center of that distribution may be taken as our best estimate of centenarian prevalence, and the sensitivity of that center to changes in the underlying assumptions can be assessed.

According to stable population theory (e.g., Keyfitz 1985), the proportion of the population above age 100 is as follows:

$$_\infty c_{100} = \int_{100}^{\infty} c(x) \, dx = \int_{100}^{\infty} b \, e^{-rx} \, l(x) \, dx$$

$$= \frac{\int_{100}^{\infty} e^{-rx} \, l(x) \, dx}{\int_{0}^{\infty} e^{-rx} \, l(x) \, dx}$$

$$= \frac{\int_{100}^{\infty} e^{-rx} \, l(x) \, dx}{\int_{0}^{y} e^{-rx} \, l(x) \, dx + \int_{y}^{\infty} e^{-rx} \, l(x) \, dx} \quad (6)$$

$$= \frac{l(y) \int_{100}^{\infty} e^{-rx} \frac{l(x)}{l(y)} \, dx}{\int_{0}^{y} e^{-rx} \, l(x) \, dx + l(y) \int_{y}^{\infty} e^{-rx} \frac{l(x)}{l(y)} \, dx}$$

where x in these integrals denotes age, b (in this equation only) is the birth rate, r is the population growth rate, $l(x)$ is the probability of survival from age 0 to x, and y is some intermediate age (in our example, age 50) such that precise mortality estimates are available only above age y. The complication of splitting the integral in the denominator at age y is necessitated by the fact that our parametric mortality model is valid for adult ages only. For convenience, we choose $y = 50$.

Lacking estimates of $l(x)$ for $x<y$, it is necessary to approximate the first integral of the denominator. Assuming a linear decline in the survival curve from age 0 to y, i.e., $l(x) = 1 - \frac{x}{y}(1 - l(y))$ it is possible to show that

$$\int_0^y e^{-rx}\, l(x)\, dx \approx l(y) \left(\frac{1 - e^{-ry} - rye^{-ry}}{r^2 y} \right) - \left(\frac{1 - e^{-ry} - ry}{r^2 y} \right) \qquad (7)$$

Using these formulas, we can calculate the prevalence of centenarians in the stable population, $_\infty c_{100}$, given three quantities: 1) the probability of surviving from age y to x, $l(x) / l(y)$, for all $x > y$; 2) the probability of surviving from birth to age y, $l(y)$; and 3) the population growth rate, r.

The values of the parameters in equation (6) were selected in a manner that reflects our uncertainty about their true values during the pre-industrial period. The result is a set of simulations where the exact values of the chosen parameters are different for each trial. First, a set of simulations were performed using a "base model". Next, various modifications to the base model were made and additional sets of simulations were computed in order to evaluate the sensitivity of the results to changes in assumptions.

For each trial, the choice of parameters for the base model can be described briefly as follows:

1. e_{50} was fixed at 14 years.
2. $_5 m_{50}$, c, and $l(50)$ were drawn at random from normal distributions whose means were chosen conditionally based on all previously selected parameters. (In other words, using the same set of high-mortality model life tables as before, the distribution for $_5 m_{50}$ was centered on the predicted value from a simple regression on e_{50}; the distribution for c was centered on the predicted value from a multiple regression on e_{50} and $_5 m_{50}$; and the distribution for $l(50)$ was centered on the predicted value from a multiple regression on e_{50}, $_5 m_{50}$, and c.) In each case, the standard error for this distribution was set equal to the maximum residual (from the respective regressions) divided by 3.
3. v was drawn at random from a normal distribution centered on 1.0, with a standard error of 0.2.
4. The population growth rate, r, was fixed at 0.05%, which equals the long-term annual growth rate of the human population during the agricultural era. (The population growth rate was not allowed to vary within each set of simulations since we can be more certain about its value, at least in the long term, than about the parameters of the mortality model.)

After choosing the parameters for each simulation trial, equation (6) was used to compute the prevalence of centenarians, expressed as a proportion of the total (stable) population. The resulting distribution of prevalence estimates is shown in

Figure 7. It is evident that these estimates have a wide range, reflecting the uncertainty about centenarian prevalence that results from our uncertainty about the relationships between the various parameters of the mortality model. After a logarithmic (base 10) transform, however, the distribution of prevalence estimates has a nearly symmetrical shape. The median prevalence estimate in the base model, as reported in Table 4, is 4.7 centenarians per 100 million population. Expressed as a base-10 logarithm, the median estimate equals -7.33 and thus lies squarely in the middle of the distribution shown in Figure 7. Although the entire distribution has a rather broad range, over three fourths of these prevalence estimates are above 1 per 100 million (or 10^{-8}).

These results provide further (and stronger) support for our earlier conclusion that centenarians must have been observed at least on occasion once world population surpassed 100 million. By our previous arguments, with e_{50} equal to 14 years, around three quarters of the plausible mortality scenarios yielded a high probability of observing at least one centenarian *every hundred years* once world population exceeded 100 million. Now, over three fourths of our plausible mortality scenarios (with e_{50} fixed at 14 years, accompanied by various age patterns of mortality) predict an average of at least one centenarian *at any given moment* out of a population of 100 million.

Table 4 also gives prevalence estimates for super-centenarians (individuals aged 110 years or older) derived from the simulations of the base model. These results suggest unmistakably that no individual was likely to have survived to age 110 during the agricultural era. The median estimate for the prevalence of super-centenarians in this model is 0.002 per 100 million. At this level, a population of 100 million persons observed for 1000 years would have only an expected 2 person-years of super-centenarian lifetime. Such a small expectation can reasonably be equated with our everyday notion of impossibility. Only the most optimistic 10-15 percent of the simulated mortality scenarios produce estimates of super-centenarian prevalence that might contradict the conclusion that there were no individuals living past age 110 during the agricultural era. Thus, although there may have been occasional centenarians for the past 4 or 5 thousand years, it appears that super-centenarians were most likely a product of the mortality decline of the industrial era.

The sensitivity of the centenarian prevalence estimates is evaluated in Table 5. This analysis varies the levels of mortality (e_{50}) as well as the other parameters of the mortality model ($_5m_{50}$, c, and v). In the former case, four additional (fixed) values of e_{50} are employed. In the latter three cases, the distributions of the simulated parameters are increased or decreased by one standard error relative to the base model.

Another sensitivity test varies the size of the standard error (σ) used in the simulations. In the base model, the standard error used for deriving $_5m_{50}$, c, and $l(50)$ equalled the maximum residual (from each regression) divided by 3. For a sensitivity analysis, a smaller σ was obtained by dividing by 4; a larger σ, by 2. Two other modifications to the base model were the "wild card $l(50)$" and variations in the population growth rate, r. For the "wild card $l(50)$" trial, the simulations were modified to include an occasional choice for $l(50)$ that was unusually high given the levels of e_{50}, $_5m_{50}$, and c (to mimic the Far Eastern mortality pattern, which was dropped from the earlier regression model of $l(50)$).[7]

Most of these changes yielded results that would not materially alter our conclusions regarding the prevalence of centenarians in pre-industrial times: for most scenarios, nearly three quarters or more of the simulations predict at least one centenarian per 100 million population. One exception to this rule is the scenario with a growth rate of 2 percent. Sustained growth rates of this magnitude in pre-industrial times must be considered very unlikely, however, so we need not be overly concerned with this result. On the other hand, it is important to examine the effects of altering the overall level of mortality (e_{50}) or the conditional distribution of $_5m_{50}$ (given e_{50}).

In each of the simulations, the level of $_5m_{50}$ was derived from a regression model (with e_{50} as the independent variable). It is clear from Table 5 that a shift of one standard error in the conditional distribution of $_5m_{50}$ has a relatively larger impact on the distribution of prevalence estimates than the other sensitivity tests, with the exception of changes in the mortality level itself (i.e., e_{50}). Nevertheless, these sensitivity tests would not alter the most important conclusion of this analysis, namely, that the expected prevalence of centenarians worldwide exceeded one well before the industrial era. Even in the scenario labeled "Lower $_5m_{50}$", three quarters of the scenarios have prevalence estimates above 0.35 per 100 million. Thus, at least one centenarian would be expected in a population of 300 million or more, which was achieved during Roman times. At the other extreme, the "Higher $_5m_{50}$" scenario suggests that a population much smaller than 100 million might have contained at least one centenarian (on average). It is difficult to argue that these scenarios are extremely unlikely: the centers of the (conditional) distributions of $_5m_{50}$ differ from the regression model by one standard error, which is only one third of the maximum residual from the regression. Thus, there remains a degree of uncertainty about the

---

[7] With a probability of 95 percent, $l(50)$ was drawn by the method of the base model. With a probability of 5 percent, the predicted value of $l(50)$ from the regression of the base model was increased by 0.2 (while retaining the same standard error).

precise timing of the emergence of centenarians, although we can remain fairly certain that the emergence (by this definition) preceded the industrial era by nearly 2000 years or more.

Obviously, it is the overall mortality level that has the largest impact on our predictions regarding the prevalence of centenarians through history. If late adult mortality was lower (e_{50} equal to 16 or 18 rather than 14 years), we might expect to see centenarians at much smaller population sizes: with more than three fourths of the prevalence estimates above 1 per 10 million, we might predict that centenarians have existed almost since the dawn of the agricultural period some 10,000 years ago. On the other hand, if late adult mortality was higher (e_{50} of 10 or 12 years), we would have difficulty claiming that the emergence of centenarians occurred prior to the mortality decline of the industrial era. Our basis for believing that agricultural e_{50} was centered around 14 years was presented in the preceding section and will not be repeated here. It is obvious, however, that the strength of our conclusions regarding the timing of the emergence of centenarians depends critically on this assumption.

Discussion

It is possible, of course, that the reality may be a mixture of the mortality scenarios we have presented here. Undoubtedly, different populations living at the same moment experienced different mortality conditions, due to variations in diet, environment, and exposure to disease. This chapter essentially ignores these spatial variations and considers what the average mortality level of the entire world population might have been. Given the absence of detailed information, this strategy seems to be a useful simplification. There appear to be no obvious theoretical reasons for worrying about the effects of heterogeneous mortality patterns on our conclusions. A more thorough investigation of this topic would perhaps be warranted but is beyond the scope of this study.

Another form of variation in mortality patterns that we have thus far dismissed may also deserve more careful consideration. Although we have argued that there is no clear evidence of a long-term temporal trend in mortality levels during the agricultural era, it seems prudent to entertain at least the possibility of such a change. For example, if there was a gradual increase in late adult life expectancies (e.g., e_{50}) during this period, then the gradual emergence of centenarians in the population might be attributed to *both* decreasing mortality *and* increasing population size. Contemplating this scenario, we might wish to restate our main conclusions regarding occasional centenarians or prevalence levels for centenarians in the population. In each case, we would define a cut-off point in terms of *both* a mortality level *and* a population size where we would expect to find some minimal level of centenarians. Using our earlier criteria (a preponderance of evidence that there would have been at least one centenarian per century, or an average of at least one living centenarian at any given time), we would seek a combination of e_{50} and total population size that would give positive indications of the emergence of centenarians. Based on the evidence presented here, one combination that would work would be an e_{50} around 14 years or greater and a population size of at least 100 million. Decreases in e_{50} would need to be associated with very large increases in population size: for example, an e_{50} around 12 years would require a population size of over 1 billion people in order to indicate the emergence of centenarians by either of our two criteria.

Finally, we may note that the two criteria for the emergence of centenarians that we have examined may seem to be rather different, and yet they produce very similar results. For example, it is obvious that a prevalence estimate indicating an expectation of one or more living centenarians at all times is a stricter requirement than a very high probability of observing at least one centenarian per century. The relationship between the two criteria is not simple, however: an expectation of one centenarian per year (on average) is by no means a guarantee of one centenarian in each single-year cohort. In fact, we know that this expectation must be around 5 or more in order to observe at least one centenarian with virtual certainty. Thus, the strictness of the two criteria differs, in some sense, by a factor of around 20, not by a factor of 100.

Why, then, do the two criteria yield similar results, if in fact one criterion is 20 times more difficult to achieve than the other? The answer lies in the operationalization of the two criteria. In effect, because it was more amenable to a simulation exercise, the prevalence criterion received a more careful operationalization. The occasional centenarian method examined a very broad range of parameters, some of which stretch the limits of plausibility, and sometimes gave equal weight to parameter choices that were not equally likely. In particular, our operationalization of the occasional centenarian method included consideration of a model assuming exponential increase in the age pattern of mortality ($v = 0$). In our quantitative summaries, we gave equal weight to this scenario, although it can not be considered equally likely based on available evidence. This choice, in particular, had the effect of making the occasional centenarian criterion more strict, thus yielding results that are similar in character to the prevalence criterion. It would of course be possible to operationalize the occasional centenarians criterion using a simulation model, but we have chosen to present the results of this method in their current form because they are informative in a different way. So presented, the results help us to understand the importance of each parameter in the mortality model. In terms of our final results, however, it is better to rely on the conclusions of the prevalence model.

Conclusion

The arguments and conclusions of this chapter can be summarized as follows:
1. Reliable records of centenarians in pre-industrial populations are not widely available. Therefore, statistical models are a useful tool for determining whether it is likely that some centenarians may have lived during the agricultural era.
2. There is no conclusive evidence of major long-term changes in human mortality levels prior to about 1600 A.D. Through most of human history, life expectancy at birth, e_0, appears to have been centered in the low to mid twenties, perhaps around 24 years. Life expectancy at age 50, e_{50}, is thought to have averaged around 14 years. These conclusions are based both on a wide range of direct evidence (see Table 1) and on two collections of model life tables (Coale-Demeny 1983, Preston *et al.* 1993).
3. Centenarians remain a rarity even in modern, low-mortality populations, with an estimated prevalence around 50-100 per million.[8] Thus, statements claiming that "centenarians were very rare prior to industrialization" do not distinguish modern from pre-modern mortality regimes in a meaningful way.
4. Nevertheless, it is possible to define arbitrary criteria that allow us to estimate the timing of the "emergence of centenarians." Two criteria of emergence are proposed here: 1) virtual certainty ($p \geq 0.99$) of at least one centenarian per century, and 2) a prevalence estimate that implies at least one living centenarian (on average) at any time. In both cases we examine a variety of plausible mortality scenarios and claim evidence of emergence if and only if

---

[8]For example, Labat and Dekneudt (1989) estimate that there were 3000 centenarians in France in 1988. Thus, in one of the world's most aged populations, numbering around 57 million, there are some 52 centenarians per million population. Similarly, there were an estimated 25,000 centenarians in the United States during 1985 (U.S. Bureau of Census 1987). In a population of some 240 million, this corresponds to a frequency slightly greater than 100 per million. Since the French population is generally more aged than the U.S. population (for example, in terms of the proportion above age 65), we should expect a higher proportion of centenarians in France than in the U.S. Although the U.S. figure is derived from Social Security records, it may still be biased upwards by age exaggeration (Coale and Kisker 1990).

a preponderance of evidence (three quarters of the scenarios) is consistent with such a conclusion.

5. Using the prevalence criterion, our best estimate indicates that the emergence of centenarians should have occurred by around 2500 B.C. in a world population of some 100 million persons. Thus, this emergence probably occurred during the time of the first great human civilizations (e.g., the Old Kingdom in Egypt, the Sumerian period in Mesopotamia). This conclusion, however, is very sensitive to our assumption about the average level of e_{50} in the pre-industrial period. Although our evaluation of the available evidence leads us to the conclusions stated here, if e_{50} was in fact nearer to 12 than to 14 years throughout this period, then Jeune's hypothesis that there were no true centenarians prior to 1800 may be closer to the truth.

6. Finally, although we believe that the emergence of centenarians probably occurred well before the industrial era, our analysis provides rather strong support for the assertion that there were almost certainly no true super-centenarians (individuals aged 110 or above) prior to the mortality decline of the past 200-300 years.

Literature

Aarssen, K., and L. de Haan. 1994. On the maximal life span of humans. *Mathematical Population Studies* 4(4):259-281.

Acsádi, G., and J. Nemeskéri. 1970. History of Human Life Span and Mortality. Budapest: *Akademiai Kiado*.

Bhat, M.P. 1987. Mortality in India: Levels, trends and patterns. Ph.D. diss., University of Pennsylvania.

Biraben, J-N. 1979. Essai sur l'évolution du nombre des hommes. *Population* 34(1):13-25.

Coale, A.J., and P. Demeny. 1983. Regional Model Life Tables and Stable Populations. New York: *Academic Press*.

Coale, A.J., and E.E. Kisker. 1990. Defects in data on old-age mortality in the United States: New procedures for calculating mortality schedules and life tables at the highest ages. *Asian and Pacific Population Forum* 4(1):1-31.

Cohen, M.N. 1989. Health and the Rise of Civilization. New Haven, Connecticut: *Yale University Press*.

Davis, K. 1951. The Population of India and Pakistan. Princeton, New Jersey: *Princeton University Press*.

Durand, J.D. 1977. Historical estimates of world population: An evaluation. *Population and Development Review* 3(3):253-296.

Flinn, M.W. 1981. The European Demographic System, 1500-1821. Baltimore, Maryland: *Johns Hopkins University Press*.

Gavrilov, L.A., and N.S. Gavrilova. 1991. The Biology of Life Span: A Quantitative Approach. New York: *Harwood*.

Gumbel, E.J. 1937. La Durée Extrême de la Vie Humaine. Paris: *Hermann*.

Gumbel, E.J. 1958. Statistics of Extremes. New York: *Columbia University Press*.

Hollingsworth, T.H. 1977. Mortality in the British peerage families since 1600. *Population* (numéro spécial):323-351.

Horiuchi, S., and A.J. Coale. 1990. Age patterns of mortality for older women: An analysis using the age-specific rate of mortality change with age. *Mathematical Population Studies* 2(4):245-267.

Horiuchi, S., and J.R. Wilmoth. 1994. Deceleration of age-related mortality increase at older ages: Testing the predictions of the heterogeneity hypothesis. Annual Meeting of the Population Association of America, Miami.

Jeune, B. 1994. Morbus Centenarius or Sanitas Longaevorum? *Population Studies of Aging # 15*, Odense University, Denmark.

Johannson, S.R., and S. Horowitz. 1986. Estimating mortality in skeletal populations: Influence of the growth rate on the interpretation of levels and trends during the transition to agriculture. *American Journal of Physical Anthropology* 71:233-50.

John, A.M. 1988. The plantation slaves of Trinidad, 1783-1816: A mathematical and demographic enquiry. Cambridge, England: *Cambridge University Press*.

Jordan, C.W. 1975. Life Contingencies. Chicago: *Society of Actuaries*.

Kannisto, V. 1988. On the survival of centenarians and the span of life. *Population Studies* 42:389-406.

Kannisto, V. 1994. Development of Oldest-Old Mortality, 1950-1990: Evidence from 28 Developed Countries. Odense, Denmark: *Odense University Press*.

Keyfitz, N. 1985. Applied Mathematical Demography. New York: *Springer-Verlag*.

Koplan, J.P. 1983. Slave mortality in nineteenth-century Grenada. *Social Science History* 7(3):311-320.

Labat, J-C., and J. Dekneudt. 1989. Combien y a-t-il de centenaires? In: INSEE (ed.), *Les Menages: Mélanges en l'honneur de Jacques Desabie*, Paris: Imprimerie Nationale.

Lee, J., C. Campbell, and W. Feng. 1993. The last emperors: An introduction to the demography of the Qing (1644-1911) imperial lineage. In: D. Reher and R. Schofield (eds.), *Old and New Methods in Historical Demography*, Oxford: Clarendon Press.

McDaniel, A. 1992. Extreme mortality in nineteenth century Africa: The case of Liberian immigrants. *Demography* 29(4):581-594.

Paine, R.R. 1989. Model life table fitting by maximum likelihood estimation: A procedure to reconstruct paleodemographic characteristics from skeletal age distributions. *American Journal of Physical Anthropology* 79:51-61.

Preston, S.H., A. McDaniel, and C. Grushka. 1993. New model life tables for high-mortality populations. *Historical Methods* 26(4):149-159.

Roberts, G.W. 1952. A life table for a West Indian slave population. *Population Studies* 5(3):238-243.

Sattenspiel, L., and H. Harpending. 1983. Stable populations and skeletal age. *American Antiquity* 48:489-98.

Thatcher, A.R. 1980. Life tables from the Stone Age to William Farr. Manuscript.

Thatcher, A.R. 1981. Centenarians. *Population Trends* 25:11-14.

Thatcher, A.R. 1992. Trends in numbers and mortality at high age in England and Wales. *Population Studies* 46:411-426.

United Nations. 1982. Model Life Tables for Developing Countries. New York:

U.S. Bureau of the Census. 1987. America's Centenarians: Data from the 1980 Census. *Current Population Reports, Series P-23, No. 153*. Washington: U.S. Government Printing Office.

Wilmoth, J., and H. Lundström. 1995. Extreme Longevity in Five Countries: Presentation of trends with special attention to issues af data quality. *European Journal of Population*, forthcoming.

Wood, J.W., G.R. Milner, H.C. Harpending, and K.M. Weiss. 1992. The osteological paradox: Problems of inferring prehistoric health from skeletal samples. *Current Anthropology* 33(4):343-370.

Yashin, A.I, J.W. Vaupel, and I.A. Iachine. 1993. A duality in aging: The equivalence of mortality models based on radically different concepts. *Population Studies of Aging #5*, Centre for Health and Social Policy, Odense University.

Zhao, Z. 1994. Long term mortality patterns in Chinese history. Manuscript (see also this monograph).

Table 1: Estimates of Life Expectancy in Various High Mortality Populations

Source		e_0	e_{50}
Acsádi & Nemeskéri (1970)			
Stone age		21.1	12.2
Copper age		28.9	10.4
Roman era		27.8	15.7
Middle ages		28.7	10.7
Thatcher (1980)			
Breslau, 1687-1691 (from Halley)		28	17
Liverpool, 1841		26	16
English Life Table No. 1, 1841		41	21
British Peerage (Hollingsworth 1977)			
Males	cc.1550-1574*	37.8	12.6
	cc.1575-1599	36.0	14.6
	cc.1600-1624	33.6	14.4
	cc.1625-1649	31.7	14.6
	cc.1650-1674	30.0	15.5
	cc.1675-1699	33.2	15.8
	cc.1700-1724	34.9	17.0
	cc.1725-1749	38.8	18.3
Females	cc.1550-1574	38.2	11.6
	cc.1575-1599	38.3	12.5
	cc.1600-1624	35.9	12.9
	cc.1625-1649	34.2	13.2
	cc.1650-1674	33.7	17.7
	cc.1675-1699	35.3	15.8
	cc.1700-1724	37.5	18.0
	cc.1725-1749	37.4	20.4
Qing Imperial Lineage, males only (Lee et al. 1993)**			
1700-09 through 1890-99		22-42 (increasing)	9.5-12.5 (steady)
Wang clan, males only (Zhao 1994)			
0-499		-	16.8
500-999		-	16.8
1000-1199		-	17.9
1200-1399		-	18.2
1400-1499		-	18.3
1500-1599		-	18.2
1600-1699		-	17.9
1700-1760		-	16.5

Table 1: Estimates of Life Expectancy in Various High Mortality Populations, continued

Source			e_0	e_{50}
Indian Life Tables (Davis 1951)				
Males		1872-1881	23.7	13.9
		1881-1891	24.6	14.3
		1891-1901	23.6	13.6
		1901-1911	22.6	14.0
		1911-1921	19.4	14.3
		1921-1931	26.9	14.3
		1931-1941	32.1	17.8
Females		1872-1881	25.6	15.0
		1881-1891	25.5	15.6
		1891-1901	24.0	14.5
		1901-1911	23.3	14.3
		1911-1921	20.9	15.0
		1921-1931	26.6	14.4
		1931-1941	31.4	18.4
Slave Populations				
Trinidad, 1783-1816 (John 1988)				
		Females	17.3	13.5
		Males	17.3	11.9
	Guyana, 1820-1832 (Roberts 1952)		22.8	11.1†
	Grenada, 1818 (Koplan 1983)		25.9	12.7
Liberian Immigrants, 1820-1843 (McDaniel 1992)‡				
Raw, Females			2.2	7.9
Raw, Males			1.7	6.6
Conditional, Females			25.8	9.6
Conditional, Males			23.9	8.3
Sweden, 1751-1760				
Males			35.6	18.8
Females			38.5	20.3

*   The life table values for British peers refer to 25-year birth cohorts, designated by "cc." followed by the birth years.

**   Numerical estimates of Qing life expectancy were extracted from graphs published by Lee et al. and therefore are presented here as a range of values with an indication of the long-term trend in parentheses.

†   The value of e_{50} for Guyanese slaves was derived by linear interpolation using the values of e_{48} and e_{54} given by Roberts (1952).

‡   For Liberian immigrants, "raw" refers to life tables computed using all deaths recorded after arrival in Liberia; "conditional" refers to life tables computed using only deaths recorded at least one year after arrival in Liberia.

Table 2: Comparison of e_0 and e_{50} in High-Mortality Model Life Tables

	Coale and Demeny			
	Female		Male	
	e_0	e_{50}	e_0	e_{50}
NORTH				
Level 1	20.0	14.7	17.6	13.2
Level 2	22.5	15.4	19.9	13.9
Level 3	25.0	16.1	22.3	14.6
Level 4	27.5	16.8	24.8	15.2
Level 5	30.0	17.5	27.2	15.9
SOUTH				
Level 1	20.0	15.5	19.9	14.8
Level 2	22.5	16.1	22.3	15.4
Level 3	25.0	16.7	24.7	16.0
Level 4	27.5	17.4	27.0	16.6
Level 5	30.0	18.0	29.3	17.1
EAST				
Level 1	20.0	14.9	17.4	14.6
Level 2	22.5	15.5	19.9	15.2
Level 3	25.0	16.1	22.4	15.7
Level 4	27.5	16.7	24.9	16.2
Level 5	30.0	17.3	27.4	16.7
WEST				
Level 1	20.0	14.3	18.0	12.7
Level 2	22.5	15.0	20.4	13.3
Level 3	25.0	15.6	22.8	14.0
Level 4	27.5	16.3	25.3	14.6
Level 5	30.0	16.9	27.7	15.2

Preston, McDaniel and Grushka		
e_0	e_{50}	
	Female	Male
10	11.3	10.0
12	11.8	10.5
14	12.3	11.0
16	12.7	11.5
18	13.2	11.9
20	13.7	12.4
22	14.2	12.9
24	14.7	13.4
26	15.2	13.9
28	15.8	14.5
30	16.3	15.1

Table 3: World Population Estimates from the Neolithic Revolution until 1750 (in millions)

Year(s)	Indifference range
10,000-8,000 B.C.	5-10
0-14 A.D.	270-330
1000	275-345
1250	350-450
1500	440-540
1750	735-805

Source: Durand (1977), Table 5.

Table 4: Simulated Estimates of the Prevalence of Centenarians and Super-Centenarians (per 100 million population)

	Percentile				
	2.5	25	50	75	97.5
Centenarians	0.099	1.30	4.72	16.9	143.5
Super-Centenarians	0	0.00025	0.00209	0.0127	0.4051

Table 5: Sensitivity of Centenarian Prevalence Estimates (per 100 million population)

	Percentile				
	2.5	**25**	**50**	**75**	**97.5**
Base model	0.10	1.30	4.72	16.9	144
$e_{50} = 10$	0.00	0.00	0.00	0.03	2.0
$e_{50} = 12$	0.00	0.05	0.31	1.7	30
$e_{50} = 16$	1.25	13.5	35.4	87.2	401
$e_{50} = 18$	8.98	66.7	155.9	324.0	1083
Higher $_5m_{50}$	0.53	7.41	26.0	79.7	610
Lower $_5m_{50}$	0.02	0.35	1.32	4.4	36
Higher c	0.03	0.69	2.71	9.5	86
Lower c	0.31	3.07	8.94	31.3	189
Higher asymptote	0.02	0.50	2.09	9.5	83
Lower asymptote	0.31	3.53	10.1	27.5	178
Larger σ	0.02	0.80	4.43	25.4	514
Smaller σ	0.23	1.73	4.81	12.2	73
Wild card l_{50}	0.10	1.32	4.82	16.5	161
$r = -1\%$	0.22	2.91	10.6	37.5	311
$r = +1\%$	0.05	0.61	2.21	8.0	69
$r = +2\%$	0.02	0.27	0.98	3.5	31

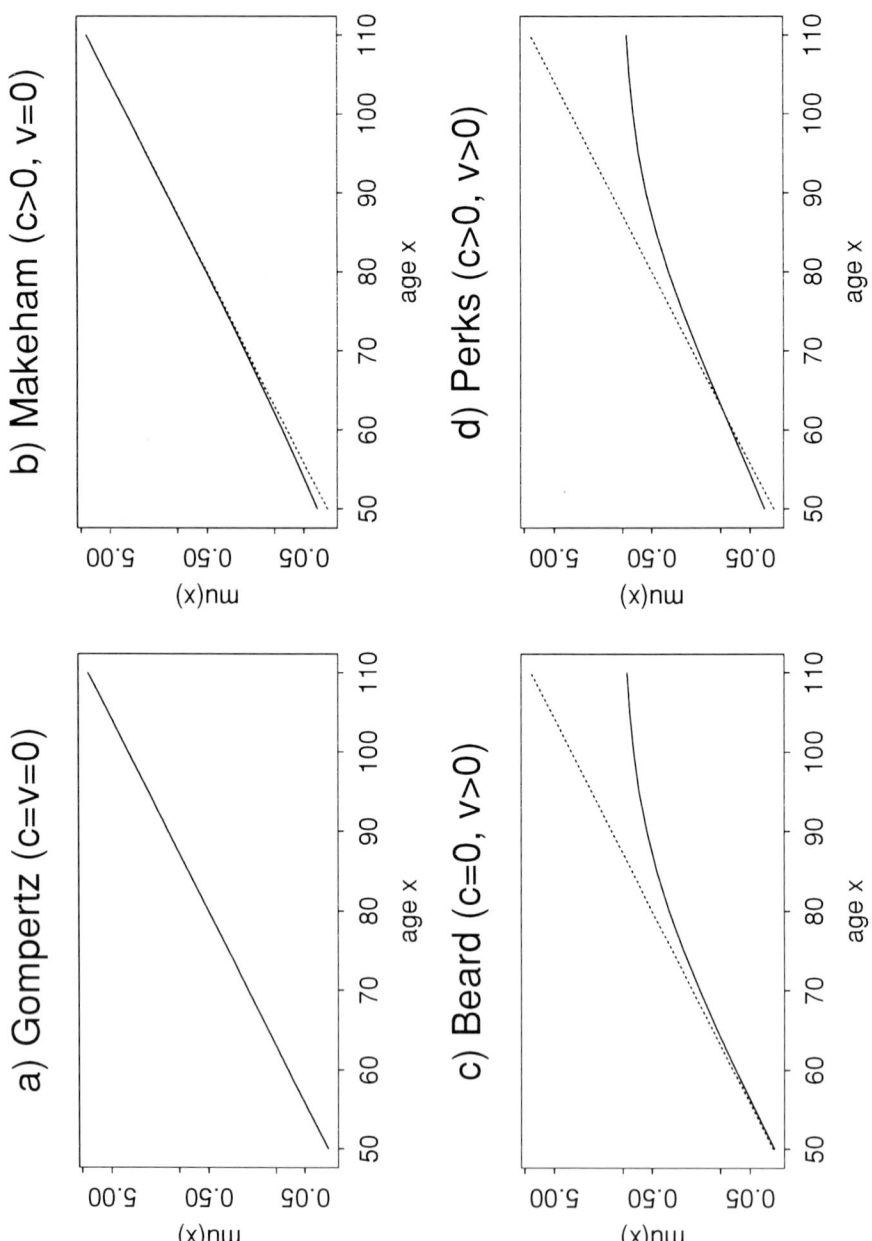

Figure 1. Gompertz-Perks Family of Mortality Curves.

Notes:
1) Parameter values used in this illustration are: $a = 0.00025$, $b = 0.095$, $c = 0.008$, and $v = 1$.
2) Dotted lines show Gompertz curve for comparison.

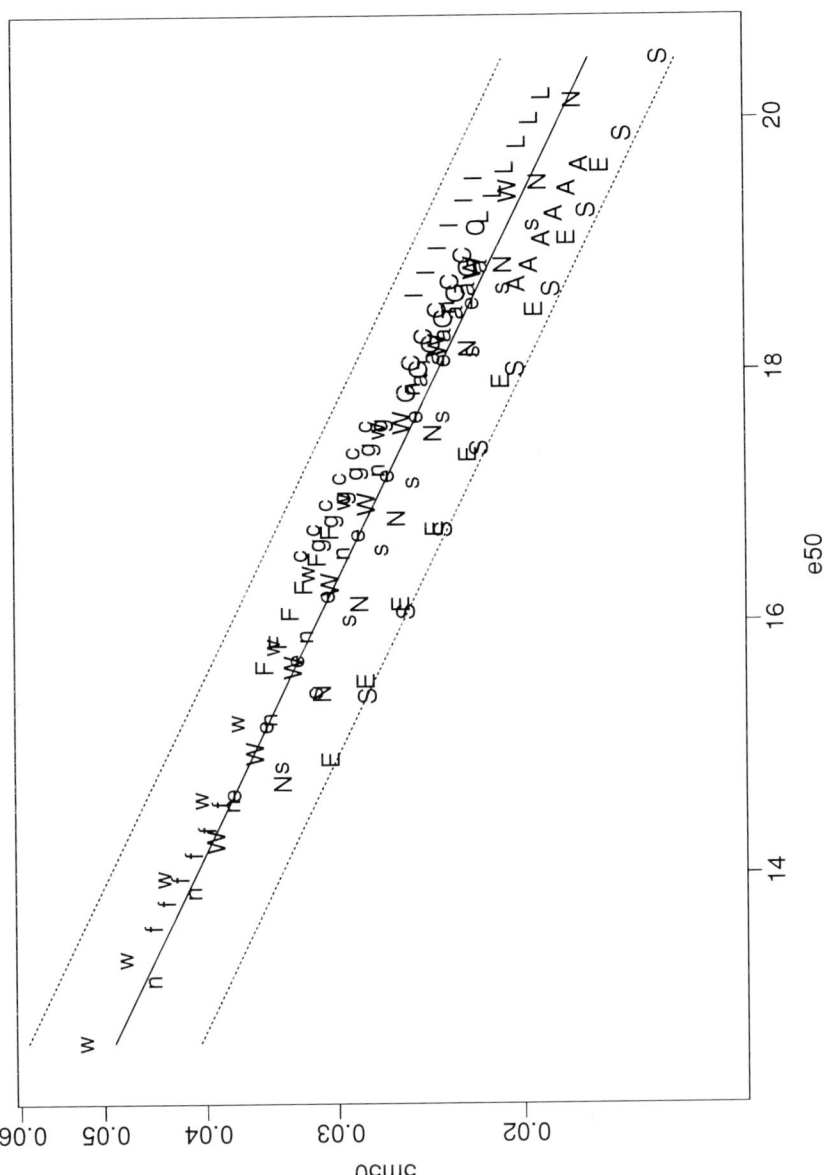

Figure 2. Relationship between e_{50} and $_5m_{50}$ in Coale-Demeny and U.N. model life tables, showing OLS regression line plus and minus its maximum residual.

Notes:
1) Logarithmic scale on Y-axis;
2) UPPER CASE = female, lower case = male;
3) E = East, N = North, S = South, W = West (Coale-Demeny);
4) C = Chilean, F = Far Eastern, L = Latin American, A = South Asian, G = General (U.N.).

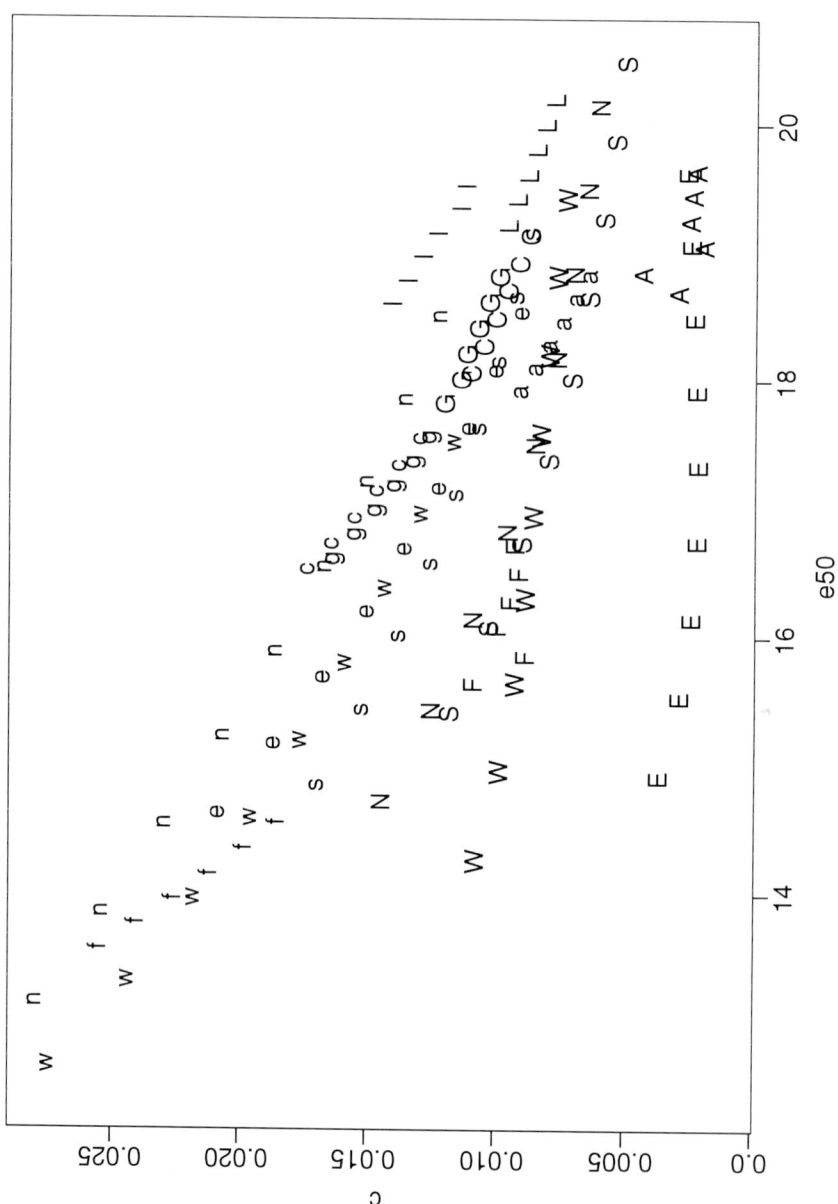

Figure 3a. Relationship between e_{50}, and c in Coale-Demeny and U.N. model life tables.

Notes:
1) UPPER CASE = female, lower case = male;
2) E = East, N = North, S = South, W = West (Coale-Demeny);
3) C = Chilean, F = Far Eastern, L = Latin American, A = South Asian, G = General (U.N.).

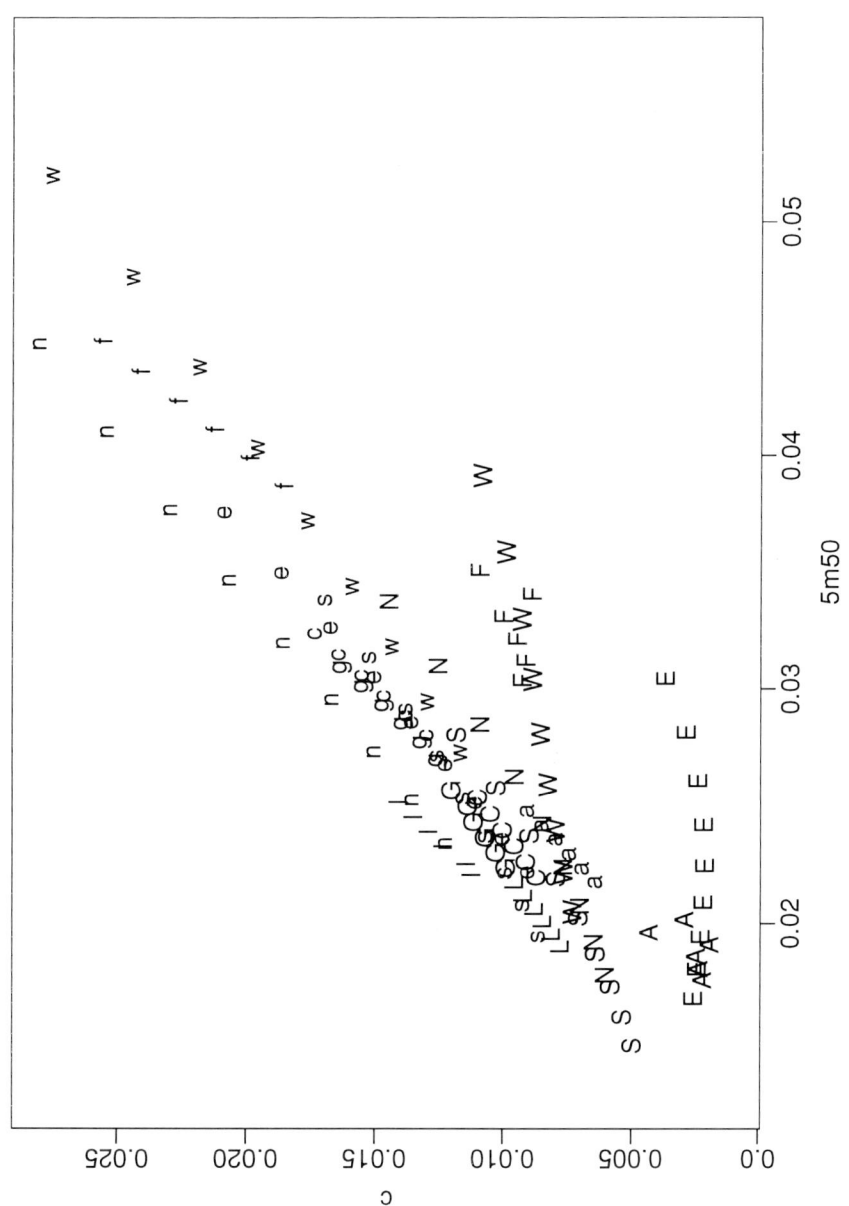

Figure 3b. Relationship between $_5m_{50}$, and c in Coale-Demeny and U.N. model life tables.

Notes:
1) UPPER CASE = female, lower case = male;
2) E = East, N = North, S = South, W = West (Coale-Demeny);
3) C = Chilean, F = Far Eastern, L = Latin American, A = South Asian, G = General (U.N.).

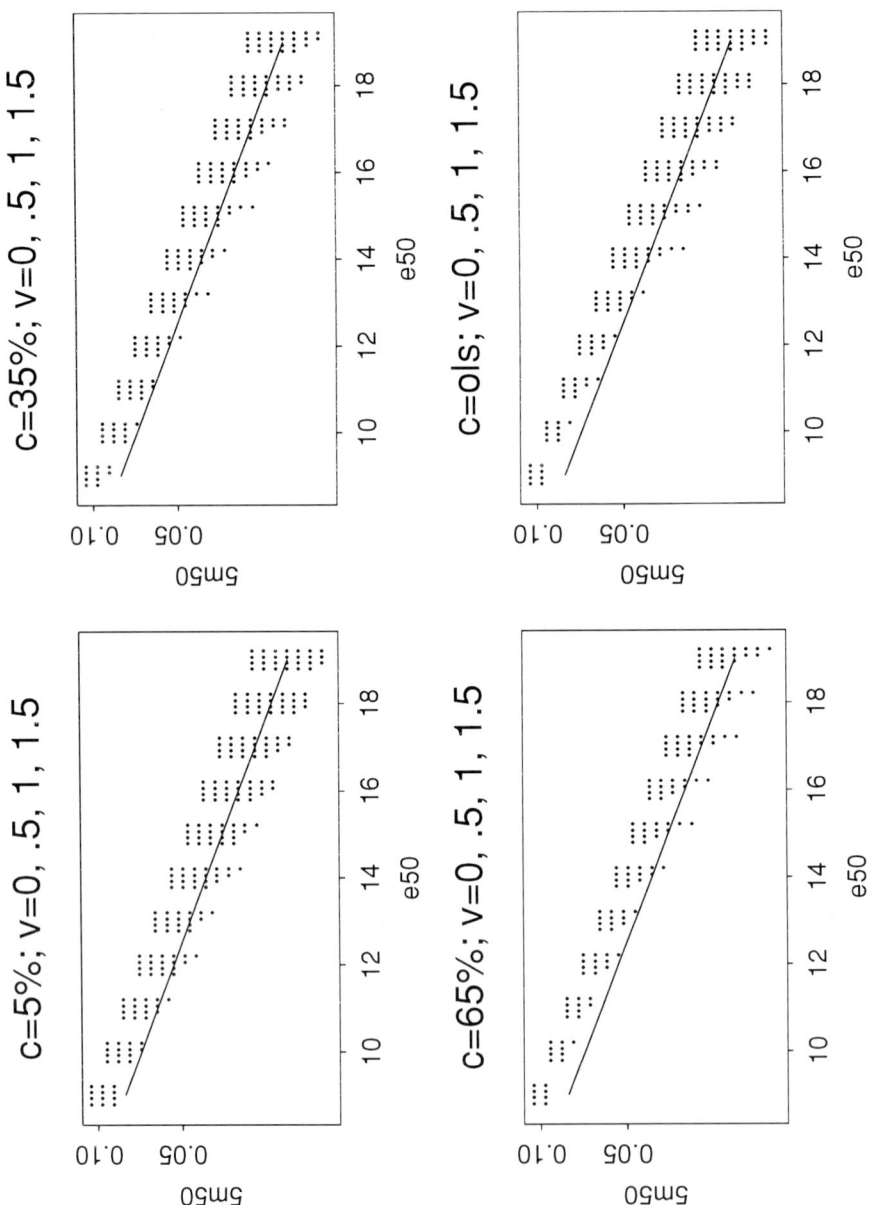

Figure 4. Hypothetical scenarios to evaluate the likelihood of observing an "occasional centenarian" circa 8000 B.C. (see text for explanation).

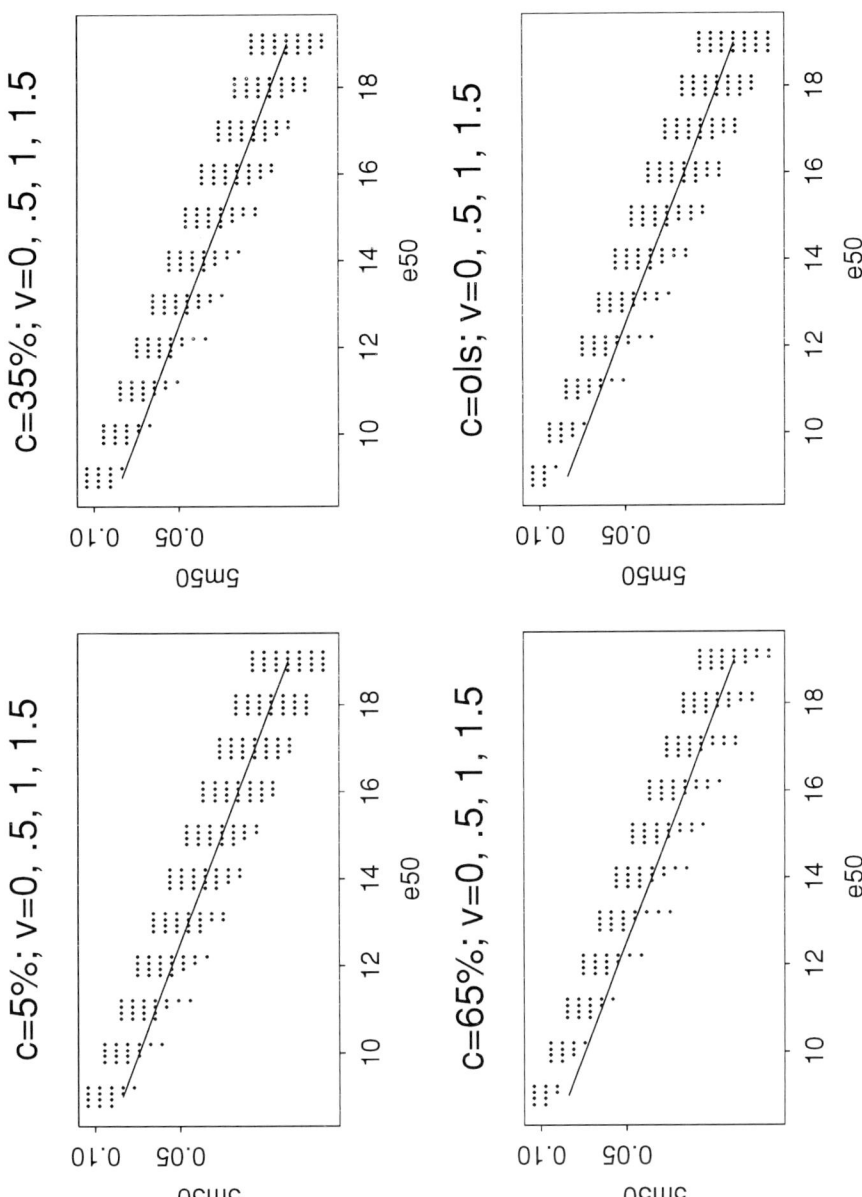

Figure 5. Hypothetical scenarios to evaluate the likelihood of observing an "occasional centenarian" circa A.D. 0-14 (see text for explanation).

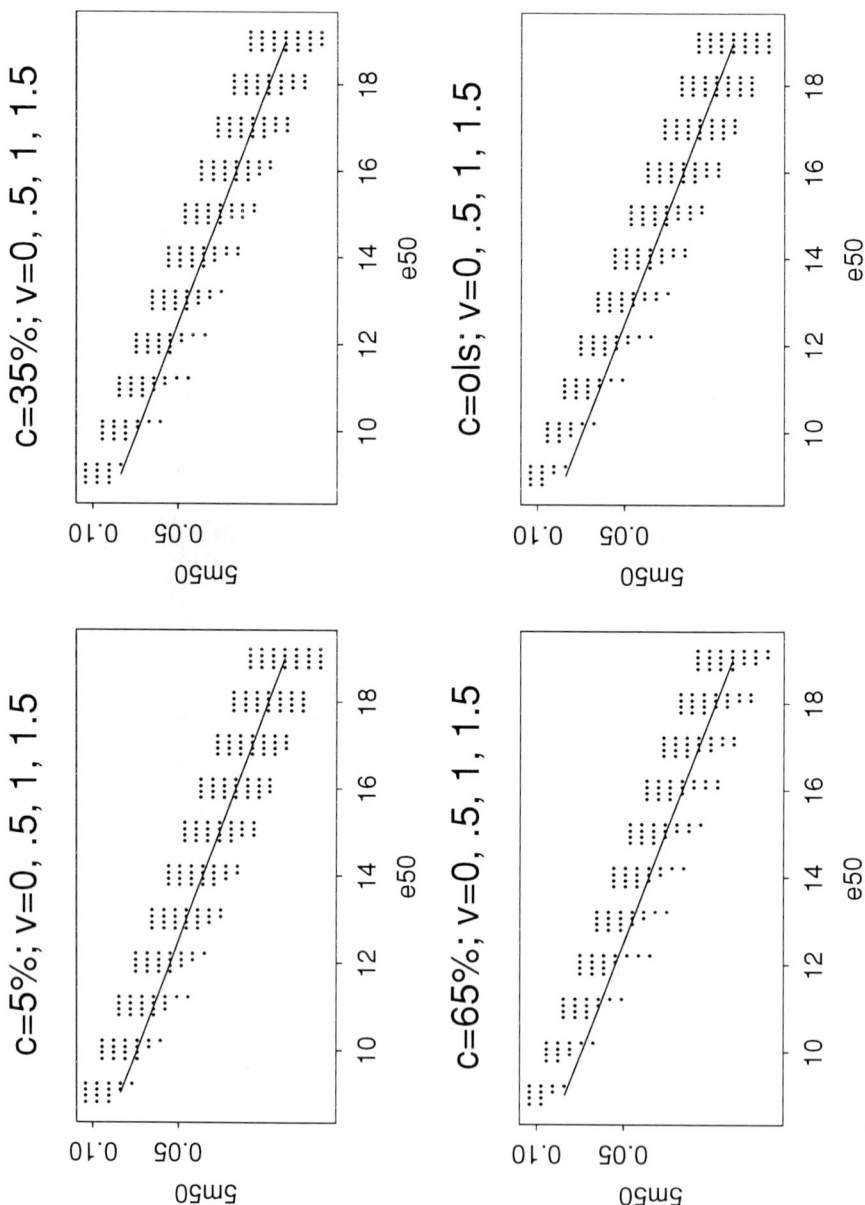

Figure 6. Hypothetical scenarios to evaluate the likelihood of observing an "occasional centenarian" during the 17th century A.D. (see text for explanation).

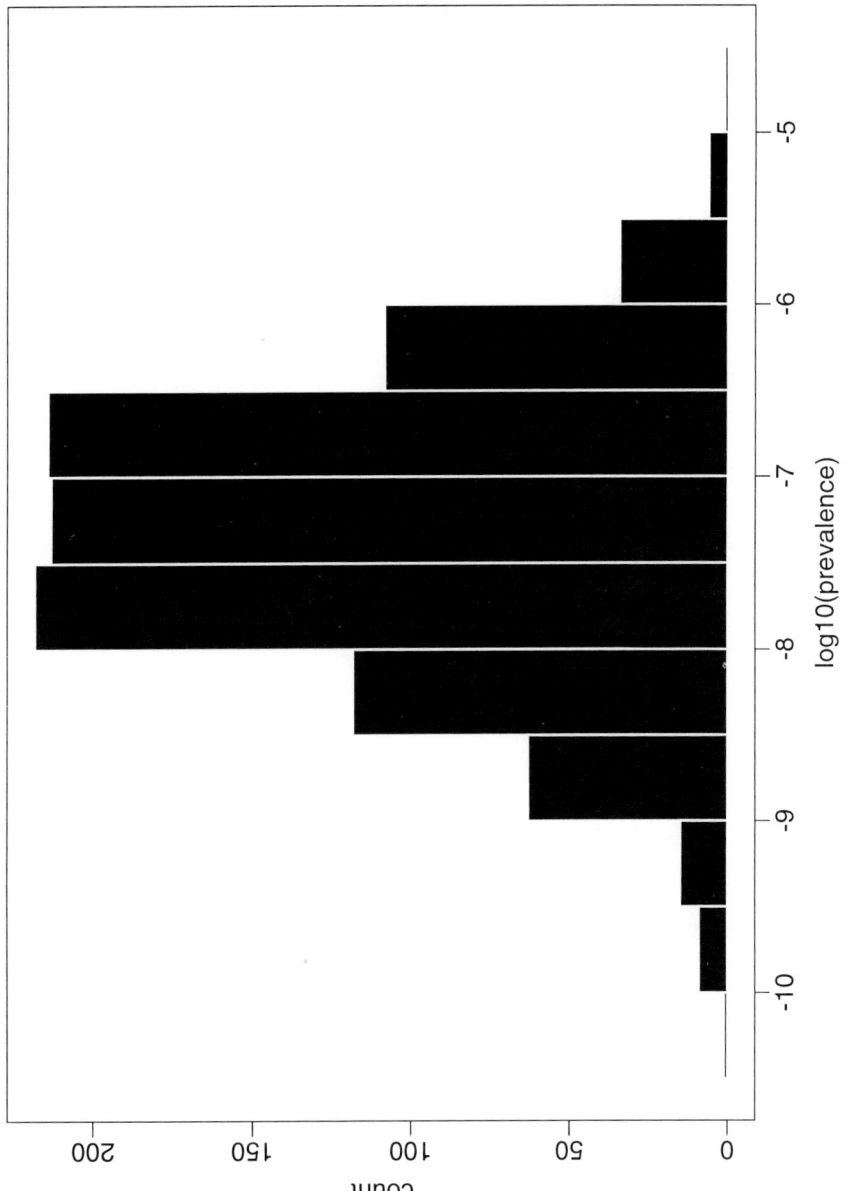

Figure 7. Histogram of simulated prevalence estimates in "base model" (see text for explanation).

Notes: Histogram shows the logarithm (base 10) of simulated prevalence estimates. The total number of estimates is 1,000.